T0167058

# The Other End of the Stethoscope

## The Physician's Perspective on the Health Care Crisis

### Diana Reed, M.D.

authorHOUSE®

*AuthorHouse*™
*1663 Liberty Drive*
*Bloomington, IN 47403*
*www.authorhouse.com*
*Phone: 1-800-839-8640*

© *2012 Diana Reed. All rights reserved.*

*No part of this book may be reproduced, stored in a retrieval system, or transmitted by any means without the written permission of the author.*

*Published by AuthorHouse 2/28/2012*

*ISBN: 978-1-4685-4412-1 (sc)*
*ISBN: 978-1-4685-4411-4 (hc)*
*ISBN: 978-1-4685-4410-7 (e)*

*Library of Congress Control Number: 2012900909*

*Any people depicted in stock imagery provided by Thinkstock are models, and such images are being used for illustrative purposes only. Certain stock imagery © Thinkstock.*

*This book is printed on acid-free paper.*

*Because of the dynamic nature of the Internet, any web addresses or links contained in this book may have changed since publication and may no longer be valid. The views expressed in this work are solely those of the author and do not necessarily reflect the views of the publisher, and the publisher hereby disclaims any responsibility for them.*

This book is dedicated to my husband Allen and to my best friend, Leslie Maschino, RN, whose support throughout times of sickness and health was immeasurable. Also a special thanks to my friend Glynis Wallace, DMD, who gave me the final push to complete and publish this work.

# CONTENTS

# FOREWORD

Leslie and I were sitting around her table when I said half-jokingly, "I should write a book about what it's really like to be a doctor in this day and age. Most people don't seem to have any idea how tough things have gotten. The glorified lives of doctors on TV are far from real life. Maybe people would understand then how difficult it is for physicians to practice, and appreciate their doctors more." Instead of laughing or belittling the idea, she encouraged me to go for it, and so this book became an eight-year-long project—a labor of love.

My purpose in writing this book was to inform and educate people about the life of a doctor, the rigorous training involved, the daily routine of medical practice, and the difficulties of reconciling the business of medicine with our ultimate goal of healing. My emphasis is on how the health-care and malpractice crises affect physicians, and on how the doctor-patient relationship has suffered. I explain how physicians cope with illness as patients. I report initial responses of physicians to the passage of the new health-care plan. And I present suggestions for solutions to the continuing problems facing doctors in this country.

I was trained in California, attending UC–Irvine for medical school and UC–San Diego for a neurology residency. I have worked in five different states, in solo private practice, small groups, large multispecialty groups, locum tenens, academic university practice, and I have been employed in radiology managed care. I had two children during medical school, and at the peak of my clinical career I became disabled. With a wide range of experience in medicine and in life's challenges, I felt that I had something to contribute to the health-care literature, especially in light of the changes coming as a result of the Patient Protection and Affordable Care Act of 2010. While there is promise of improving access to health care for patients, the burdens placed on physicians and their attitudes toward this legislation need to be discussed. We need to understand the issues from the physicians' perspective—from the other end of the stethoscope.

The contents of this book reflect my opinions and experiences, except where supported by surveys of physicians, statistics or specific references.

My mission is to convey the importance for all people to pay attention to the medical profession, to understand their physicians' struggles and rewards, and to assist in salvaging the relationship between doctor and patient, which is suffering. I hope this book helps to promote better communication and transparency in the medical field. My advice to those of you considering a career in medicine or surgery is to go into it with open eyes and an open heart. For the rest of you—humanity—please remember that physicians too are only human.

# The Physician

My healing hands
Are tied
By loopholes,
Knotted by lawyers,
Bound by insurance or
Lack thereof.

Would that I could
Give it all up, but
This calling is strong.
I was created
To serve.
Every day
I rise above
The frustration.

To experience
The joy of healing
Is my life's purpose.

# INTRODUCTION

Do you think doctors have it made? When you get sick and need a doctor in the middle of the night, do you take for granted that doctors will always be available to care for you? Would you want to be a doctor in this day and age? Why are we losing good doctors to early retirement and other careers?

Most people are aware that there is a health-care crisis in America. However, few have examined the crisis from a physician's point of view. The general public, the government, and insurance companies are mainly concerned with the cost and availability of medical care. How these issues are affecting America's doctors is a mystery to most people. Few people have insight into the daily struggles that physicians face in the twenty-first century while trying to provide excellent care to their patients. People seem to have forgotten that physicians are the foundation of health care, and without them there would be no one to administer treatment, perform surgery, or interpret results for disease or trauma.

A huge number of physicians in private practice have dropped out, many seeking alternative careers because of rising job dissatisfaction. In this book, I hope to enlighten readers about the physician's life and how the current medical climate has affected everything we do, every decision we make, and our career satisfaction. The long and rigorous training involved in becoming a physician changes us in ways we never dreamed possible. The interactions with patients that make up our days can be difficult and rewarding, as well as intense and stressful. The doctor-patient relationship has deteriorated and is fraught with mistrust from both ends of the stethoscope. If we are to turn the current situation around, we must understand the issues.

In this book, I will discuss the difficulties involved in the business of medicine and the gradual loss of the private-practice model as huge conglomerate health-care corporations take over this country's delivery of medical care. Finally, I will provide a perspective on the future of physicians and medical care in America. I will make some suggestions on how patients and physicians can work together to reverse some of the trends that are hurting health care in America.

Every living person should have concerns about health care. If you sit in a public place and listen to the conversations of people around you, the subject eventually turns to health problems that they or someone they know are having. People used to complain that their doctors acted as if they thought they were God. Nowadays, people seem to expect their doctors to be gods—perfect in their diagnosis and treatments and able to predict the future. When the physician fails to live up to those expectations, as they inevitably do, since they are human, patients often see this as a reason to sue. Many people use an illness with a poor outcome as a chance to win millions of dollars in awards from "jackpot juries" in the litigation lottery. The people on these juries often feel sorry for the injured parties, but this doesn't mean there is always negligence on the part of the physicians. Lawyers also try to increase their odds of winning a verdict by suing everyone involved in the patient's care. If successful, the lawyers get to keep an average of one third of the award for themselves. It's no wonder the number of malpractice claims —and insurance rates—are increasing dramatically every year.

Many people imagine their doctors living a life of leisure and luxury. They have no idea of the sacrifices doctors make in their personal lives from the time they enter medical school until they retire. They are not aware of the thirty-six-hour shifts most physicians endure, or the long and unpredictable hours of each workday. There are also difficulties being successful in the business of medicine, for which most doctors are poorly prepared. In addition, there are huge amounts of paperwork required for each patient seen and frequent battles with insurance companies to get approval for tests or medicines for their patients. Constantly changing billing requirements and regulations by the government and insurance companies often leave many bills unpaid. While the costs of operating a private practice are increasing exponentially, reimbursements are going down every year. Because of this mismatch, physicians are pressured to see more patients each day, packing their schedules in order to survive financially. This is one of the only businesses in which practitioners are not paid what they charge, but what the government and insurance companies decide to pay. Because of laws that prohibit collective bargaining, physicians have no bargaining power, and our only choice is whether or not to be a provider for a given insurance plan. If we choose not to be providers, this means fewer patients walk in our doors. Refusing to treat patients because of their insurance type goes against our ethical and moral principles; the Hippocratic Oath to provide care to all people as we see the need, not a hypocritical oath for wealth care instead of health care.

When people go to their doctor, they expect the doctor's undivided attention, and they should expect to be listened to, diagnosed, and treated with both compassion and competence. However, many diverse patients are seen in a given day. A physician's day involves caring for the very young and the very old, the poor and the wealthy, the uneducated and the highly trained professional. We may see routine medical problems as well as life-threatening emergencies in any given day and often find ourselves pulled in many different directions as we try to prioritize our time. Generally, patients have an expectation of perfection in diagnosis and treatment, and they often have unrealistic expectations of a cure that physicians are incapable of providing. There is increasing suspicion and cynicism among patients that erodes the trust upon which the doctor-patient relationship is built. This and the rising malpractice climate have led to the practice of "defensive medicine," which is increasing the cost of medical care without increasing its quality. When every patient with a headache gets a $2,000 MRI of the brain, everyone pays in rising insurance costs and taxes. At the same time, when a physician begins to see every patient as a potential lawsuit that could end his or her career, ordering unnecessary tests to rule out rare or unlikely causes of a patient's symptoms is a matter of self-preservation.

We are trained and motivated to provide the highest quality medical care to all of our patients, to consider their welfare above all else, and to do no harm. People should understand that there is an emotional, human aspect to physicians—despite their encyclopedic knowledge of medicine they need spiritual gratification from their work and it is this spiritual reward above all others that drives physicians to sacrifice so much to serve others. The current system is designed to stratify health care and puts the doctor in the uncomfortable position of doling out medicines, tests, surgery, and life-changing treatments according to insurance company benefits or lack of insurance coverage. Physicians have become conflicted and morale has gradually worsened because of our inability to reconcile the practice and the business aspects of health care in the current system.

I hope to shed some light on the arduous journey one makes going from college graduate to physician in the longest training program of any profession. Despite all the difficulties, most physicians choose a career in medicine not for monetary rewards, but because of the deep, unconditional love and empathy we have for our fellow humans, scientific curiosity, and the emotional and spiritual rewards of healing and helping our patients cope with illness. However, most physicians today are unhappy with their careers. According to recent statistics, more than half of practicing physicians in America would not recommend a career in medicine to their children or friends. The respect, trust, and dignity that used to be integral to a physician's life have been all but lost, in favor of a computerized, big-business atmosphere where both physicians and patients feel as though they are rushed through their visit, and the human interaction is lost in the shuffle. The long-term relationships that physicians and patients enjoyed over years—even generations—are gone, as people switch doctors repeatedly because of changes in their insurance plans. As a result, many physicians seek alternate careers due to job dissatisfaction. Older physicians are retiring early in huge numbers (The Physicians Foundation). Several health related groups now predict a tremendous shortage of physicians in the years to come (Federal Advisory Group Predicts Physician Shortage Looming).

The sacred relationship between doctor and patient has been so deeply eroded that one might question whether the basic trust that is so integral to the healing process can be salvaged. We need to change as a society and improve access to health care for all Americans, make health-care insurance affordable for employers and individuals alike, and control the runaway costs of the pharmaceutical companies, litigation, insurance companies, and managed-care corporations. We need to see our physicians not just as expensive commodities in health care or adversaries, but as our friends and partners in the battle against disease. We also need to accept that some people get sick and die, despite the best efforts of their physicians. We need to realize that physicians are human, and, like everyone, they are subject to make occasional mistakes no matter how they may strive toward perfection. Many of the top doctors in the country have the longest records of malpractice lawsuits. Many of them work in teaching hospitals where they not only train the new generation of physicians but also care for a large percentage of the poor and uninsured. These are some of the best physicians in the world, and they should not be measured by the lawyer's yardstick.

For the amount of time, sacrifice, and stress physicians undergo each day on their jobs, should they not make a good living? Health-care expenses are not the highest in the world because of physicians' salaries, but because of other factors like pharmaceuticals, hospitals, insurance companies, and legal costs. Powerful corporations and their lobbyists have tight control over the political system and are strongly motivated to maintain the status quo, which is providing them with record profits, while sucking the life out of small businesses and individuals, who are struggling to pay record-high medical bills.

In these troubling times, I hope this book will help afford some insight into the lives of physicians and their struggles, to foster better understanding, communication, and compassion so that we can work together to heal the medical system that affects us all. If you are considering a career in medicine, you owe it to yourself to get a better understanding of the daily struggles you will face as a physician, as well as the joys of caring for and helping people to get well. I hope that the book will shed some light on the realities of a career in medicine and help strengthen the resolve of at least a few premed students to choose this most challenging way of life with their eyes and their hearts open. Being a physician is one of the most challenging careers that exists, and you will learn new things and meet all kinds of memorable people throughout your career. You must be prepared, however, to overcome the frustrations of paperwork, the risks of liability, and your own inadequacies in order to find satisfaction as a physician in this time of uncertainty in health care today. You will need to take an active role in helping to shape the future of medicine so that the most important aspects of medicine are not lost. Patients and physicians need to understand each other more fully, to see things from both ends of the stethoscope, if we are to bring about badly needed changes in our health care system.

# CHAPTER 1:
# A CAREER IN MEDICINE

A career in medicine used to be viewed as one of the highest callings anyone could have—it was seen as a noble profession associated with respect, appreciation, and trust. Being a physician was regarded as one of the best things a person could do with his or her life. Medical schools were able to recruit the best and brightest students from college, and acceptance to medical school was extremely competitive. Aspiring physicians were some of the most intelligent and idealistic people, filled with enthusiasm about the opportunity to heal others and to learn everything they could about the human body, illness, and treatments. Is the medical field still a noble profession?

I grew up in the sixties and seventies, a rebellious era for most young people. My father died of lung cancer when I was sixteen, and his death shut me down emotionally for a long time. Because I was such a bad student and always in trouble, I dropped out of public high school and went to a free school called Skunk Hollow High School. Needless to say, I was not voted most likely to succeed, nor was I the class valedictorian or a cheerleader. In fact, no one would have pegged me as a future neurologist, yet from these nontraditional roots, I stumbled into this noble career. Skunk Hollow High School was a place filled with hippies, musicians, artists, and philosophers. There were no grades, no scheduled classes, and no attendance taken—basically no rules. At a time when I was rebelling against everything remotely authoritarian and struggling to define myself as a young teen, I finally found myself in a place where there was nothing to rebel against. I have many great memories associated with this school, but the greatest lesson I learned in this midst of true academic freedom was that unless you got up and did something with your life, nothing happened. If I wanted to learn something, I had to find the teacher or resource and make it happen. If I wanted to be good at something, I had to learn the discipline of practicing, studying, and hard work. This has been a cornerstone of my philosophy of life, and I admit I often have difficulty understanding those that wait their whole lives for something to happen or for someone else to make decisions for their futures. I became interested in herbs and nutrition, perhaps as a reaction to the failure of traditional medicine to heal my father's cancer. It was my first inkling of something that would consume my life. Perhaps it was a way to take control of an event over which I had no control.

After high school graduation, I moved out to California in my little white VW van, piano in the back, boyfriend in the front, and all the world ahead of me, undiscovered. I played the French horn to the cows at rest stops along the way. I enrolled in the local college to take a few courses that interested me while I worked days as a file clerk in a court reporting office. Anatomy and physiology, psychology, microbiology, and Edible Wild Plants comprised my first year's schedule. By the end of the year, I was hooked on learning about the human body. I became more and more aware of how little I really knew. I then took a course in deep tissue massage that incorporated principles of healing, movement, and energy analysis—alternatives to traditional medicine—which were highly controversial. I experienced the joy of touching others, experiencing their energy, and making a difference in how they felt. I was learning to develop my perception of others, looking for blockages in their energy fields or auras, and to channel my own energy to heal others.

As my knowledge of health and illness grew, I came to realize that there are basically two kinds of patients. There are those with mild ailments that are not life-threatening, often associated with physical or emotional stress, musculoskeletal aches and pains, or depression. Many of these people can get tremendous benefit from healing massage, acupuncture, or chiropractic treatment. In addition, nutrition and herbal remedies often help minor ailments and generally improve health. There is, however, another group of people who have much more serious illnesses that are frequently life-threatening, who are in need of "real" doctors. I found myself wanting to be the real doctor, to have the knowledge and ability to deal with the serious illnesses that affect peoples' lives. For better or for worse, I decided that I wanted to know more, to do more and to help more sick people, and so I became a premed student. I completed my bachelor's degree in chemistry. I took the MCAT exams. My mother, who was a singer and assistant professor of music, was surprised that I would give up my budding career as a french horn player to pursue medicine. I remember telling her that I just couldn't see myself tooting in the back of the orchestra for the rest of my life. Although I was never voted most likely to succeed, I became determined to reach for the top with a career in medicine.

## RECRUITING THE BEST AND THE BRIGHTEST

Getting into medical school used to be extremely competitive, and only those with the highest GPAs, MCAT scores, and demonstrable interpersonal skills were accepted from thousands of applicants each year. Applicants had to show that they had some experience in a health-related field, or excellent accomplishments, in addition to grades and test scores, that made them a better person. For example, an applicant had to have good communication skills, especially the ability to listen. He or she should have a track record of service to others. Demonstrated leadership ability was a plus. And most important, did the individual's behavior show a consistent pattern of compassion, honesty, and altruism —character traits that are consistent with the highest standards of professionalism?

It took me two tries to get accepted into medical school. The first rejection was a big blow, and I realized how poorly prepared I was, as well as how little I knew about the medical field. I took the MCAT exam a second time, improving my scores, and spent a year as a research technician in a lab run by a hematologist/oncologist who was working on a cure for melanoma, a particularly deadly form of cancer. After the first rejection, it was very tough to get the courage and confidence to try again for a medical career, but fortunately the people around me did not let me give up. I knew so very little about what being a doctor was really like. Working with a physician in his lab helped open my eyes to the difficulties of treating diseases like cancer that had no cure, with limited treatments available. Before this, I guess I had an idealistic notion that I would spend the majority of my day making brilliant diagnoses and being showered with love and gratitude from adoring patients. I certainly didn't believe I would end up like my uncle, who was a general practitioner in the New York City projects, treating underprivileged and frequently ungrateful patients most of the day in a small, dingy, office that smelled of antiseptic and old age. I didn't think much of his situation when I decided to go into medicine, but now, as I look back, he was perhaps one of the most honorable professionals I ever knew.

While acceptance into medical school is still competitive, many of the best and brightest students are choosing other careers after learning about the difficulties that doctors face today. Medical school applications are down in numbers (FACTS: Applicants), and many of the brightest students are opting for careers with greater financial rewards and lower demands. Who in their right minds would want to deal with training that consumes half of one's life, followed by the actual job that is incredibly demanding and time-consuming, all for a shrinking income and rising overhead? I recently met a young man in high school who told me he was planning to become a neurologist, like me. It was all I could do to encourage him in his efforts. I had to hold my tongue when I thought of all the challenges he would face in pursuing a career in medicine. I knew that he had no idea what demands, disappointments, and sacrifices his choice would entail on a daily basis.

Most premed students have very little idea of what is involved in the practice of medicine. Getting into medical school is just the first of many hurdles to overcome.

## INDOCTRINATION OF MEDICAL STUDENTS

Medical school entails four years of intense study after completion of a bachelor's degree. After completion of medical school, a residency is required that may involve another three to seven years, depending on the specialty one chooses. By the end of medical school, students are now called "Doctor," but they are still woefully unprepared for the practice of medicine. Residency turns them into seasoned, well-trained professionals, but many choose to stay in training for another one to two years for a fellowship, in order to concentrate on a subspecialty. Sometime in their late twenties or thirties, physicians can finally embark on their careers. Most are excited about going out and tackling what is considered by many to be the most challenging occupation that exists. Little do they know how challenging this career will be and the types of obstacles they will encounter while trying to provide the best quality care for their patients.

The process one goes through in medical school is a very complex combination of intense study and test taking, introduction to patient care, and learning to interact with patients in a nurturing way. By developing the ability to question and examine patients, formulate differential diagnoses, order the appropriate tests and confirm our final diagnoses, medical students become medical detectives. Once a diagnosis is confirmed, we can then choose a treatment that is most likely to be effective, which may involve medication, surgery, or the many other options available today to treat disease. This involves a great deal of science, as well as intuition. There are many individual patient factors involved in choosing the appropriate treatment for a given illness, such as coexisting illnesses, drug interactions and insurance plans. There are also many psychological factors involved in the art of medicine that require a physician to interact with their patients in a supportive and educational role.

I spent the first two years of medical school in classrooms, reading thousand-page books, taking tests, and dissecting the dearly departed who had the courage to donate their bodies to medical science. I remember my first day in the anatomy lab. It seemed like yesterday that I was having some difficulty dissecting frogs without gagging, and suddenly I was surrounded by dead human beings. Most of us were praying that we wouldn't throw up or pass out. We uncovered these stark, naked, aged bodies that had been preserved in formaldehyde, wrinkled and frightening—just shells of former souls that once walked the earth. At the same time, we had a tremendous sense of appreciation for these men and women who had donated their bodies so medical students could learn. We honed our skills in dissection and surgery on these cadavers as we prepared ourselves to work on the living. After a month, we became desensitized to the sights and smells of the anatomy lab. A driving curiosity and motivation took over as we cut and dissected limbs, chests, brains, faces, and eyes. Our exams consisted of pins stuck in various muscles, nerves, arteries or veins with questions about the pinned structure. This was just the beginning of our transformation into physicians. We were also studying physiology, biochemistry, pathology, and pharmacology, just for starters. These basic sciences were the foundation for the many aspects of human health and disease we would be learning over the next several years.

Medical school was an incredibly rigorous and demanding training that required hours of study both in and out of the classroom. The goal was perfection, to know it all, which could never be achieved. This didn't stop us from striving for it. There were many long nights spent cramming for exams, and many times I felt that I could not cram another fact into my head. I wondered often during those first few years whether I would ever be worthy of being called "Doctor." When one of my fellow second-year medical students committed suicide, the rest of us began to realize the degree of stress with which we were all struggling, and that this was only the beginning of our careers. She was one of the best students in our class, usually getting the top scores on exams. Underneath that incredible genius, however, was an emotionally fragile young woman, and none of us recognized her anguish. Evidently, she was not able to deal with the inner demons we all had lurking under the surface. We began to realize then that perfection was impossible, that knowing it all was impossible, and that mistakes would be made, some of which would affect human lives. We had to accept our imperfections and do the best we could. There have been recent articles focusing on the problem of medical student depression and suicidal ideation, which is a far more common problem than ever previously recognized (Dyrbye et al., 2008). Fortunately, shedding light on such an issue helps all of us cope with those feelings and realize we are not alone in the tremendous emotional upheaval we are experiencing. It also may help friends to recognize when a fellow student is in trouble and needs our help. The transformation from Joe the college grad to Dr. Joe, the surgeon, is not a simple one.

The second half of medical school is the clinical portion. We were finally allowed to enter the hospital with our starched, short, white coats (the long coats were only allowed for the real doctors). At first it was a challenge just to find our way around the hospital, the lab, X-ray, and then to find our "team." The team was made up of attending physicians (the teachers that ultimately supervised the patient's care), the residents (physicians in training for their specialty), and the medical students (the bottom rung of the ladder). It seemed that everyone in the hospital knew more than we did about the practical aspects of patient care, including the nurses.

We were assigned a few patients about whom we were to learn everything. We quickly found out how little we knew, despite the past two years of intense study. We were useful to the team mainly in obtaining results of tests, keeping track of our patients' vital signs, and attempting to present those results on daily rounds. Scut monkey is the endearing term for medical students on a team and playing that role was an initiation rite that we all went through. If you did your job without griping, went home and studied the diseases of your patients and the meanings of those test results, you were rewarded with pearls of knowledge the residents would share, when time allowed.

We followed our residents around like loyal puppy dogs, trying to emulate their behaviors with patients without showing our ignorance. We could not write orders, we could not make any medical decisions regarding our patients, and we weren't much help on the team except for that scut work that saved our residents some time. We were apprentices, learning the art of taking histories and doing physicals, learning diagnosis and differential diagnosis, the appropriate tests to order, and treatment options for disease. We learned about death and dying, a true lesson in humility for a future healer. We learned about birth, and in the process we were reborn ourselves.

I still vividly remember the first time I saw a patient die during my gynecology rotation. She was very old and had suffered with ovarian cancer. I observed as my senior resident came into the room and spoke with the family. The family members shed many tears, and I was crying too, even though I did not know this patient. It was the first time I had been so close to death since the death of my own father years before. My resident was not crying, however, and I wondered at the time how she maintained her composure. After we left the room, she kindly took me aside and assured me that these situations would get easier in the future. I prayed that she was right, yet I wondered what was happening to my humanity. Was I losing it or was I just being trained to withhold my emotions to benefit my patients? Was my ability to empathize with my patients and their families enhanced or diminished? Later, since I became a neurologist, I've had many family meetings at the ends of my patients' lives. I learned so much by observing my residents and attending physicians interacting with patients and their families, that there are no textbooks or even words for. I am grateful every day for the opportunity to have experienced the moments when I saw the miracle of healing in action, even at the end of life. This was the motivation and the true reward that kept me going day after day.

Our patients knew we were just medical students and not real doctors and often felt put upon at a time when they were under tremendous stress. We would spend two or three hours on our histories and physicals, which patients in a teaching hospital often endure multiple times during their stay. As we learned to do procedures, the patients allowed us students to practice on them. It was not always a pretty sight, as we struggled with spinal taps, arterial blood gases and learning to put needles accurately in the bodies of our patients for various tests and treatments. I am so thankful for the Veterans Administration and university hospital patients, who stoically tolerated my early attempts to learn the skills necessary to become a physician. There was one old man at the VA who put up with me attempting to draw a blood gas from the radial artery in his wrist multiple times before I got the hang of it. He must have been in severe pain, yet he never let on. I suppose on some level he enjoyed the attention he got from all the med students, and compared to fighting in a war, perhaps this was not so bad. Yet even to this day I think of him and remember the kindness of an old vet who donated his body to science, even in life.

We took call in the hospital with our team every third or fourth night. We would be up all night on many of those call nights, seeing patients who came in through the emergency room and those already in the hospital who were having problems. This was our first introduction to the thirty-six-hour days we would experience about twice a week during residency. There's nothing like lying in the call room—usually a converted patient room or closet—with a single bed with hospital sheets and blankets that reeked of the hospital Laundromat, and a cheap little alarm clock, phone, and pad of paper ready to take the next call. Inevitably, it is just as you get off to sleep that the beeper goes off. You turn on the light, and as your eyes adjust, you peer at the number. Two AM? Of course, it's the ER. The bright, wide-awake ER doc begins to tell you about the patient they are seeing and asks would you come take a look, as you sit up and throw on your shoes and white coat. You throw a little water on your face, and off you go. A couple of hours later, you may get to try again for some sleep. It is such a wonderful experience that many of us wrote poems or songs or skits about those good old days, which we would perform at our graduations. I wrote one song while I was on call titled "Sittin' in La Jolla VA" to the tune of "The Dock of the Bay" by Otis Redding.

Sleep became a luxury we were often deprived of, though we tried to appear fresh and clear-minded as we presented our patients' cases on morning rounds. Since I completed my training, legislation has been passed to cut down on resident physicians' on-call hours because of the large numbers of mistakes made by sleepy residents. It took several years of lobbying to get people to recognize that human beings, even physicians, cannot function well without sleep. There are no such regulations for practicing physicians, however, and it is common for physicians to work eighty to one hundred hours per week.

During the third year of medical school, we rotated through ten-week blocks of the major specialties—internal medicine, general surgery, obstetrics and gynecology, psychiatry, and family practice. Most of the time was involved in caring for hospitalized patients. During the fourth year, we were exposed to some medical specialties such as cardiology, emergency medicine, neurology, orthopedic surgery, and ophthalmology. We worked in outpatient clinics. We had elective time to choose rotations we were leaning toward for our own careers. We were overwhelmed by the knowledge and skills of our residents and attending physicians, and by our own inadequacies. What we learned during these intense blocks of time barely scratched the surface of the knowledge and skills necessary to practice these specialties. I remember holding retractors in the operating room to allow visibility into a body cavity for hours as I watched my senior residents and attending physicians perform major surgery. It was an awesome experience, even if my arms almost fell off. We were reminded continually of how much we had to learn before we could call ourselves "Doctor."

"Pimping" is another endearing term for the questioning of medical students about their patients, diseases, and treatments. This was usually done at six or seven AM on daily rounds, a meeting of the team where all the patients were discussed and treatment plans formulated. For a medical student, rounds could be a humiliating experience. Our lack of knowledge and misconceptions were fully exposed. We were evaluated and graded by the residents and attending physicians on our team, based on these interactions, in addition to the three-hour exams at the end of each rotation. Being unprepared for morning rounds was to be avoided at all costs, and being tired was no excuse. We only needed to remind ourselves that people's lives were at stake. It was impossible to be fully prepared with the limited time and knowledge we had. However, as time went by, we gradually developed our clinical skills. We practiced differential diagnosis, where a set of symptoms becomes a list of all possible diagnoses, from all possible causes, from autoimmune to vascular. Then one by one, the list is narrowed down by the clinical characteristics, the exam, lab and radiologic findings, and statistical likelihood of a given disease. Finally, in a complex whittling process of ruling out diagnoses on the list, a final diagnosis is reached. A treatment is selected based on the disease, the patient's history of allergies or other medications, and what their insurance will cover. Our reward came when our patients got well and went home. Our patients' diseases determined much of our curriculum, and most of us remember a specific patient who taught us about a specific disease. I remember the twelve-year-old middle school cheerleader who taught me about Sydenham's chorea, a rare movement disorder in children that can occur after a Strep infection. I remember the eighty-year-old retired teacher who contracted Jacob Creutzfeld Disease, caused by a virus-like protein particle that infects the brain and leads to dementia. I remember many of my Parkinson's patients, stroke patients, migraine patients, and although I can't give you their names, they have a special place in my heart and in my mind. When I am asked if a particular symptom or sign is associated with a particular disease, I think back not only to my reading, but to the patients with that disease whom I have etched into the pages of my personal history. We got to see firsthand what it was like to work in different specialties, and how different personalities were more suited to each field. Adrenaline junkies with strong type A personalities tended toward emergency medicine or critical care, while introspective, philosophical types were more apt to choose specialties like psychiatry. Those who loved the technical skills and procedures involved in medicine gravitated toward surgery. Some decided at some point they really didn't like dealing with people directly and went into pathology or radiology. The diversity of personalities helped to ensure that a broad range of medical specialties would be represented by a graduating class of medical students. In those days, the majority, however, chose primary care residencies like pediatrics, family or internal medicine.

In addition to the long hours in the hospital directly caring for our patients, we continued to study and discuss journal articles with the most recent research on their condition. There were never enough hours in the day to keep up with all the demands of training to become a competent, well-rounded physician who was up to date on all the latest research in any one field, not to mention all of medicine.

In the fall of the fourth year of medical school, we had to choose which specialty we wanted to pursue. Choosing a specialty becomes a necessity for most physicians because there is simply too much information in each area of medicine for anyone to know it all. Even family practice and internal medicine are specialties that narrow down the information required to practice. In fact, there is too much information to learn even within just one specialty. Medicine is expanding exponentially in all areas simultaneously, and many physicians end up as subspecialists, continuing their training in fellowships after residency for another year or more. Overall, the completion of a physician's training takes fourteen years or more after high school. One must be driven by long-term goals to succeed in the field of medicine and plan ahead in three- to six-year blocks of time.

What specialty a medical student chooses is often determined by a combination of factors unique to each individual. Some may have known since before medical school that orthopedic surgery was to be their chosen field. Others find a mentor during medical school who inspires them to pursue family medicine, for example. Yet others find that they have certain talents like delicate, steady hands to perform microsurgery in a field like ophthalmology. There is a vast difference in the day-to-day activities and patient interactions each specialty of medicine involves, and yet, we get very brief, if any, exposure to many specialties during medical school.

Medical school is not cheap. Most people who complete medical school usually incur huge student loan debts, and many of these debts (ironically called "HEAL loans") accumulate interest while residency is underway. The specialty one chooses and the location where they practice will affect how quickly they will be able to pay back their loans. Most residents in their final year of training were over $50,000 in debt from student loans, and many were up to $200,000 in debt, according to a recent survey by Merritt, Hawkins and Associates (2003). I was thirty-five years old by the time I finished my residency as a neurologist and $100,000 in debt. Although I was invited to stay on at the university to teach and to do research, I could not afford to do so because of the massive student loans I had incurred. The salary for university faculty is far less than that of a private practice physician. Years later, I was still paying off those student loans, as one would a mortgage on a house. For many, the choice of residency type is not based on the love of a certain field but is a financial decision, as the disparity of incomes various physicians earn becomes apparent. Most medical school graduates are choosing specialties rather than primary care in part because the salaries they can expect to earn are significantly higher. In 1998, 54 per cent of medical school graduates chose a career in primary care, as compared to 18 per cent in 2010 (American College of Physicians, 2010).

Fourth-year medical students usually have very limited exposure to the various specialties and subspecialties and little knowledge of the practical realities of those specialties. However, they choose a career that seems to be the best fit for their personality and apply for residency positions in a complex selection process called "The Match." After interviews and test scores with prospective training programs, a giant computer program integrates first, second, and third choices of the students and the medical schools. The computer then comes up with the best matches possible for each student and residency program. I felt very lucky to be accepted by my first choice in the match—Mercy Hospital in San Diego for internship and neurology residency at UC–San Diego. Many of my friends found themselves in programs that they didn't really want but were committed to accept by The Match contract agreement. Some did not match anywhere and had to scramble for the remaining unfilled positions afterward.

I chose to specialize in neurology for several reasons. From my earliest memories, I was fascinated by the brain and behavior. The dean of my medical school was a neurologist specializing in multiple sclerosis. He was a strong influence on me and incredibly intelligent, solving complex clinical diagnoses like a Sherlock Holmes of the medical field. Neurologists always got the cases nobody else could figure out, and Dr. VanDen Noort had an encyclopedic mind with a gentle, kind heart that his patients adored. He was an inspiration, not only to me but to hundreds of medical students passing through his medical school year after year.

Anyway, what organ in the body could be more interesting and challenging than the brain? The three main specialties that deal with the brain are neurosurgery, psychiatry, and neurology. I wanted to do neurosurgery, but it required a minimum of seven years of residency, and being on call was so stressful and long, I could forget about having a home life. My babies were one and three at the time, and I knew I would never see them if I picked a surgical residency. Psychiatry seemed like such a nebulous field to me and required dealing with people who were mentally but not physically ill. Neurology seemed like the perfect fit—a very challenging field that was undergoing dramatic changes and breakthroughs in diagnosis, imaging and treatment.

There are more residencies available than there are graduating medical students. Due to the rising need for physicians in all specialties, foreign medical graduates fill approximately 25 percent of these programs. For the physician who immigrates to the United States, a coveted spot in a good residency program is the opportunity of a lifetime. However, the nature of medical training across the world is very different and frequently less stringent than in U.S. medical schools, especially in the basic sciences. Many residency positions go unfilled each year. As our baby-boomer generation ages, there will be many more elderly people with medical needs. We as a nation face a predicted shortage of physicians in the future, and this may become a crisis that could take years to resolve. Considering the time it takes to complete medical training, it is important to consider the public health issues of supply and demand for physicians in our country and around the world. It is also important to keep our physicians satisfied in their careers so that they continue working, since the cost and duration of training a physician is so large. Physicians are often seen as a commodity in discussions about health care. If so, how do we as a nation preserve and protect this group that we so badly need? How do we foster the notion that a medical career is worthwhile and rewarding, and that primary care is as worthwhile an occupation as surgery?

## INTERNSHIP, RESIDENCY, AND FELLOWSHIP

In June of each year a class of medical students graduates and walks down the aisle, receiving the doctoral hood with great ceremony. They recite and swear to an oath for doctors of medicine, which is based on the Hippocratic Oath. Part of the oath I took stated, "I see my ability to be a good physician as a gift to be shared with humanity." Just when they think the worst is over, these graduates head out to begin their internship. This is the first year of training after medical school, when you are finally called "Doctor." It is considered to be one of the most stressful years of a physician's life. We looked forward to even longer hours in the hospital, carrying a beeper that went off many times per hour, day and night. Even more stressful was the increased level of responsibility, as we wrote orders and rushed to patients' bedsides for various emergencies. We were performing more new procedures and interacting directly with our patients and their families. We struggled with explaining in lay terms the condition and prognosis of our patients, based on our limited experience. I remember well the first time a patient died on my watch. It was my first night on call. I had received a checkout list from the other interns of about twenty patients I was responsible for during the night. I was asleep in the call room when the beeper went off. The floor nurse paged me about two AM to come up and pronounce a patient dead. As I tried to wake up, I struggled to understand. If she knew the patient was dead, why did she need me? He was a Do Not Resuscitate patient, and no CPR was needed. Nevertheless, I walked to the patient's room and beheld a gruesome sight. The patient had died of a cancer that had eaten away parts of his nose, mouth, and cheek. His eyes were open and had the dull stare of the cadavers we were dissecting just a few years before. I quickly put my stethoscope to his chest, listening for breath sounds. I felt his neck for a pulse, and there was none. I noted the time and walked out to the nurses' station. "He's dead, all right. Now what do I do?" I asked of the nurse on duty. With a sigh, she walked me through the protocol—as she had probably done a hundred times before with each new crop of interns—of notifying the family and documenting the time of death in the patient's chart. I thanked the nurse for the lesson learned and went back to bed. The closet-sized call room with disinfectant-smelling sheets on a hard twin bed was a welcome sight. There were no tears this time, and sleep came easily to my exhausted mind. Another lesson in becoming a physician was learned. Catch sleep whenever and wherever you can. Let go of the dead; there's nothing you can do for them. Be prepared for the next emergency, and try to keep those who are still living, alive.

As the years of residency went by, half of our lives were spent training in the hospitals and clinics. Upon completion, we could finally work in our respective specialties and begin our careers. We could prepare for the most important exam of our careers—the board certification exam. This grueling exam usually takes two days and includes written and oral portions, as well as a faculty-observed patient examination. To pass these exams, one must prepare for months. Not to pass is unthinkable, yet only a little more than half pass on their first try, and many take the boards up to three times before they succeed in becoming board certified in their chosen specialty.

As the residency comes to an end, it is time to make major life choices about where we will practice, what type of practice we want, and whether we will be independent or salaried employees. The only problem is that, despite our extensive training in medicine, most of us have had no formal business training. Most physicians have no idea what the business of medicine is like when they complete their residencies, how to read contracts, or what income or overhead to expect. The 2003 Merritt, Hawkins and Associates survey of final-year medical residents revealed that only 2 percent felt well prepared for the business side of their medical careers, 51 percent felt somewhat prepared, and 47 percent felt unprepared. Forty six percent had no formal training regarding employment issues (Merritt, Hawkins and Associates, 2003). According to this recent survey, 71 percent of graduating residents joined single-specialty groups or partnerships, very few went into multi-specialty groups (13 percent) or HMOs (1 percent), and a few (only 4 percent of the 2003 graduates) went into solo private practice. Of the major concerns these residents listed in the survey, malpractice was at the top of the list (62 percent), and managed care was second (60 percent). Other concerns raised included availability of free time, educational debt, and insufficient medical knowledge. This represents a major change from prior surveys done every two years since 1995, when concerns about malpractice and managed care were 3 percent and 14 percent, respectively. A staggering 24% stated that they would not choose a medical career if they had their education to start over.

I was filled with anticipation as my residency came to a close. I was finally going to be able to get a real job, at the age of thirty-five. I was going to pay off all my debts, including the $100,000 "mortgage" on my training. I was interviewing with neurology groups who promised what sounded like great salaries with eventual partnerships. I interviewed with hospitals that were willing to sponsor a neurologist to practice in their communities. I did not realize that every offer had a catch. There were restrictions written in to each offer that could come back to haunt me if things didn't work out. The private groups had noncompete clauses that would keep me from practicing in the area if I left the group. The hospital-sponsored programs required that I stay for a period of four to five years in order to be forgiven the debt of start-up funds. Everyone seemed to want a piece of me that they could control.

Then I met a female neurologist in solo practice who wanted to move to Colorado and needed someone to take over her practice. She wanted no money for her practice, but for me to take over her leases and contracts. Her office was somewhat small and plain, but affordable. The local hospital was willing to provide some start-up funds with the conditions that I stay three years. It sounded like the opportunity of a lifetime. I knew nothing about running a business, but if this other woman had been able to handle it, why couldn't I?

I inherited this solo private practice right out of residency. I didn't know the first thing about how to manage a practice, but with a little guidance and encouragement, I jumped in with both head and heart. Mostly heart. I hired an office manager who knew how to set up the billing and collections and run a medical office. I then found a great nurse, who had retired from the navy. I signed every insurance contract that came across my desk without even reading them. I tried to read them, but they were written in legal language, and my eyes would grow heavy as my thoughts would drift off the page. The thrill of practicing medicine, the challenge of treating my patients without supervision, without discussing them with an entire team, the responsibilities of being the "attending physician"—these were the thoughts that consumed me. I figured that if I was a good enough physician, the business would work out. As I hung out my shingle on the office door and got a goldfish for the waiting room, I started the new career for which I had spent the last fourteen years preparing.

## What Makes a Great Physician?

What makes a good or even a great physician? Perhaps it is the ability to integrate all the accumulated science and knowledge with a personality that nurtures, educates, and helps each patient feel that he or she is special and gives them hope. It is important that patients believe that they are going to benefit from their doctor's interventions. A great physician is able to foster a relationship of trust and open communication, to listen and to maintain a nonjudgmental attitude toward patients from all walks of life. Good physicians leave their own personal issues aside and place their consciousness inside of their patient's bodies and minds, conveying their knowledge and skills to allow for the miracle of healing to occur. At the beginning of medical school, I remember the dean of the medical school telling my freshman class that we were more idealistic at that time than we would ever be in our careers, and I couldn't understand what he meant. All I knew was that I was incredibly excited about having gotten into medical school. I prayed that I was up to the task of becoming a good physician. I looked forward to a career of healing and sharing my compassion, empathy, knowledge, and skills with each patient I met. I wanted to know everything there was to know about medicine and to put that knowledge to good use in healing all my patients. I vowed that I would never lose that idealism, no matter what was to come. While I admit that my idealism has been shaken up over the years, I still believe in the virtue and integrity of a medical career. There is little else that will get you out of bed at four in the morning to head to the emergency room than the principles of honor that drove us into the medical field in the first place.

Some of the top doctors in the country as rated by various surveys are those who teach and have clinical research interests and, of course, great bedside manners. They often devote a significant portion of their practices to providing care to the poor and uninsured. They are always learning more and keeping up on the latest medical news related to their specialty and applying this information to their patients. They can translate Medical-ese into normal English and communicate well with their patients. While all young physicians aspire to these goals, few are able to achieve such a delicate balance during their careers.

## MEDICINE VS. FAMILY

And what became of our personal lives while all this was going on? Friends and family often lost patience with our refusals to go out to parties or family reunions. It was hard just to be home without locking ourselves in a room to study or sleep. Our social lives became more and more limited. As our medical vocabulary grew, we had less and less to talk about besides the latest surgery we had observed, an interesting patient we had seen, or some other aspect of our training. We were often accused of speaking a foreign language. It was harder for our friends and families to relate to us, except when it came to asking for medical advice regarding their own or a family member's medical condition. They would get that glazed look in their eyes as we would attempt to explain the pathophysiology of a disease or the differential diagnosis. As a result, we tended to become more and more isolated in our so-called ivory towers. There were our fellow physicians, and there were the lay people, who comprised everyone else. We learned to speak a different language with each group. A metamorphosis was taking place that would affect our very identities as regular human beings.

Some of us tried to do the things the rest of the world were doing, like having families. I had two children during medical school, though I'm still not sure how I managed. It seemed like I wasn't home enough to get pregnant, not to mention nursing my babies or raising them. I was something of a freak, carting that pregnant belly around the medical school. When my fellow medical students held a baby shower for me, I received some very odd gifts, like rubber gloves and surgical masks for changing diapers; a pediatric textbook so I could worry more than most new parents about each fever or cough. The nurses on the maternity ward were shocked and dismayed when I brought my books to the hospital to study for upcoming final exams right after delivering my first child early in December of my second year. I brought my daughter with me to class a few times, nursing her in the back of the lecture hall as I tried to concentrate on my professors, who were teaching physiology and pathology. I was eight months pregnant again with my son when I rotated through the Ob-Gyn service. The patients whose babies I delivered certainly knew that I could relate to them. When one of our patients came into the hospital with a stillborn fetus, my heart broke for her. All the fears expectant mothers normally experience are often magnified by too much knowledge of exactly how many things can go wrong. Perhaps this is in part why doctors and nurses often make the worst patients.

By the time my second child was born, I had my fellow medical students help with my C-section, which I scheduled at the beginning of my senior vacation. This was rather controversial at a time when most obstetricians recommended trying for an unscheduled natural birth. After my vacation time was up, it was very hard to leave my babies and head back to medical school. I struggled to find day care for extended hours, and I missed my kids desperately every third night, which I spent on call in the hospital. I put a lot of pressure on my husband to pick up the pieces I left behind. As my children grew, and my professional responsibilities increased, it became more and more difficult to juggle my time without dropping the ball. I found myself rushing to pick the kids up from day care and carry them back to the hospital to finish doing rounds on all of my patients. I would leave them in the doctor's lounge unsupervised, eating hospital food, while I worked. Sometimes, I got back to find them fighting with each other or tearing the doctor's lounge apart, jumping off the chairs, playing with the TV controls, and all without any adult supervision. I admit that my kids were pretty unruly at times, and it's no wonder. I often got peculiar looks from both my professional colleagues and other mothers. I didn't seem to fit in completely with either group, and yet I was a part of both worlds. I still lie in bed at night and wonder whether I made a mistake thinking I could have it all, or whether I should have skipped one or the other aspect of my life. I think most physicians deal with a lot of guilt about the neglected spouses and children they left behind each day to give their medical careers first priority in their lives. It was a trade-off we all hoped would be worthwhile in the long run. I think many physicians nowadays question that assumption and long for the time that was lost—time that we weren't there to nurture our personal relationships and social lives. It's not difficult at times to resent our duties as physicians when we have to leave our families behind. I believe it is harder for women physicians than their male counterparts to leave children in others' care. It is hard to find men who are willing to take on a nurturing, caretaker role in the family without feeling that their manhood is somehow threatened. It is often hard for men to accept when their careers must take a backseat to their wives'. Like many physicians' marriages, my first marriage ended in divorce. In the battle of Medicine vs. Family, loyalty to my career evidently won, and family took a backseat to this all-encompassing, time-consuming vocation.

Thus begins the second half of a physician's life. As medical training—and the relatively sheltered atmosphere of our residencies—end, we take on the greatest responsibilities of our lives, making decisions day after day that are literally life or death for our patients and our careers. There is no one to report to, no one to ask questions of or with whom to confirm our diagnoses, no backup anymore. We have each been transformed from normal happy-go-lucky youths into driven, dedicated physicians, taking the world of medicine upon our shoulders.

## OATH FOR DOCTORS OF MEDICINE
Written by the University of California Irvine Class of 1977

I solemnly promise, as a physician, to practice my profession to the best of my ability. I will use my knowledge and skills to aid in the prevention, diagnosis and treatment of medical diseases. I will try to help my patients to understand disease, treatment and prognosis. I will encourage my patients to participate in decisions relating to their lives.

I will endeavor to alleviate their fears, and recognize that occasionally the most meaningful treatment may be to listen with kindness and understanding.

I will treat my patients with dignity and will give to them the respect and privacy which I would hope to receive if I were ill. I will keep their trust and preserve confidentiality. I will understand that a patient's sense of self-esteem is essential to good health.

I will value life even as I must also strive to understand the process of dying.

I will respect the wisdom of my teachers and will share my knowledge with others. I will strive to further my education and develop habits that promote further intellectual growth.

I will be proud to practice medicine to the best of my ability and humble enough to call for assistance when necessary. I will encourage and cooperate with all others involved in the care of my patients so that others can perform their duties effectively and with consideration.

I will live and practice medicine for people rather than for things. I desire that my empathy will never be subservient to skill and knowledge. I see my ability to be a good physician as a gift to be shared with humanity.

# CHAPTER 2:
## THE PRACTICE OF MEDICINE

## A LACK OF PRACTICAL EXPERIENCE

As physicians complete their training and begin their careers, they are enthusiastic and pretty well prepared for the practice of their medical specialty. They are not as well prepared for the business of medicine or the day-to-day responsibilities that have little to do with patient care. They quickly learn that the demands on their time from their patients, colleagues, insurance companies, and the government can be overwhelming. Being on call is different in private practice than it is during residency, and while most physicians take call outside the hospital, the hours are still long and unpredictable. One finds oneself driving back and forth to the hospital at odd hours to see patients from the ER or to do urgent consults. However, despite all these inconveniences, most physicians grow to love the practice of medicine. There are no words to describe the incredible feeling of satisfaction and accomplishment we have when we are able to put our training and knowledge to good use and help our patients get well. We come to feel as if our patients are our extended family, and we watch over them as a parent would watch over their children. In physician satisfaction surveys, the single most important factor that makes this incredibly difficult job worthwhile is the interaction we have with our patients (Kaiser Family Foundation, 2002). When we see the appreciation in our patient's eyes, we are gratified beyond any financial reimbursement. There are those special patients who take the time to bake a cake, or remember us at Christmastime. I have an embroidered picture from a former patient that reads, "Diana Reed MD, My Doctor My Friend," that was given to me by a particularly difficult patient. I treasure this handmade gift and have kept it up on the wall for years now. The patient who gave me this gift had been in a car accident and had a chronic pain syndrome for which treatment was challenging and for which I never received payment from the auto insurance company. I had several thousand dollars tied up in this patient's care and ended up writing off almost all of it. I had set this patient up on a payment plan of $5.00 per month, which she paid faithfully, sometimes even paying $10.00 per month. After a year of payments, I finally sent her a note forgiving her remaining debt, since, at that rate, she would have been sending me a check for twenty years. It was more of a hassle for me to keep track of the paperwork than it was worth, and I knew it was a strain on her, especially with the new disability she suffered. I don't know if it was really all that altruistic to write off her debt, but in these days when many physicians turn all their late accounts over to professional collection agencies that have no mercy when it comes to individual situations, I was proud, although poorer, for having dealt with most of my collections issues personally.

Physicians need to feel appreciated and to feel that we are respected in our communities. To know that we have sacrificed all those years for a worthwhile purpose is what keeps physicians going. It is certainly not about the money we make. That can be obtained much more easily and in greater abundance with many other ventures. When you look at a minimum of twelve years of secondary education, an average of $100,000 of student loan debt and the time involved every day to practice medicine, what person in his or her right mind would choose this career, unless there was a reward greater than money to look forward to?

## THE THREE *A*'S OF A GOOD PHYSICIAN

When I first started out as a neurologist, one of my colleagues taught me the three most important qualities of a successful consultant. These "golden rules" apply to most physicians in practice. The three *A*'s are Availability, Affability, and Ability, in that order. One should always be available and willing to see a patient when requested, regardless of the hour or extenuating circumstances. Being easily accessible builds your practice and encourages repeated consultations from referring physicians. They want to know they can count on you to see their patients, whenever the need arises.

In addition, one must always be affable, friendly, and enthusiastic with referring physicians, even when the ER is calling at two AM. I always make it a point to thank the referring physician for each consult, knowing that referrals mean work, and work is a matter of survival. One should always try to be kind and compassionate to patients and their families, who are stressed out, frequently agitated, and difficult to deal with. One should also be considerate and kind to the staff at the hospital, even when they page you in the middle of the night by accident or for an issue that could have waited till morning. A good consultant does not criticize the referring physician for any oversights or speak ill of them to the patient or their family.

When a person visits their doctor, they are often intimidated, afraid to ask questions, and frequently withhold vital information regarding their medical conditions. They may forget most of what was discussed during their visit because of this "white coat" anxiety. Physicians need to remember to allow their patients to tell their story, however. Often, as a patient begins to describe their symptoms, they are interrupted with a barrage of questions that often direct the physician down the wrong path in the diagnostic process. Listening to our patients will often lead to the correct diagnosis. My neurology teachers used to say that the history of the present illness was 90 percent of the diagnosis. This kind of interaction takes time, though, and physicians are increasingly pressured to hurry up, to ask only the pertinent questions they believe are relevant to the primary symptom. Often we end up jumping to a diagnostic conclusion that may be incorrect in our rush to see as many patients as we can each day.

People seem to forget that physicians are compassionate human beings first and foremost; our calling in life is to help them to get well. We want to establish strong, trusting, and interactive relationships with our patients. Good communication between doctor and patient is the key to accurate diagnosis and effective treatment. We measure our success in terms of good outcomes for our patients, even though good outcomes are not always attainable. However, like everyone else, we have bills to pay, personal lives, good days and bad days, physical and psychological problems and, yes, we make mistakes. We know that our mistakes can mean life or death to our patients, which adds another level of stress that few other professionals experience. With the rising incidence of malpractice lawsuits, our mistakes can also mean life or death to our careers. These concerns have made it increasingly difficult to practice medicine today.

Finally, one must have the ability to answer the questions raised by the referring physician and take over that aspect of the patient's care that is within one's specialty. This involves doing a history and physical, writing and dictating a consultation note, writing appropriate orders, performing surgery or procedures, and following up on tests and treatments that will benefit the patient. When the patient leaves the hospital, the consultant should schedule a follow-up appointment in the office. Once you accept that patient into your practice, you are responsible for them even after they go home. These guidelines constitute a code most physicians live by. We don't usually complain about these requirements; this is the nature of our careers in medicine. We don't usually express our personal frustrations to our patients or referring physicians; we leave our personal lives behind when we devote our full attention to our patients. For the most part, this physician's code is a good thing. Our patients take precedence over everything else going on in our lives. In another way, perhaps this has helped to contribute to the crisis in health care. Insurance companies, the government, and the general public take advantage of our willingness to maintain such time-consuming, highly ethical standards.

## A TYPICAL DAY IN THE LIFE OF A DOCTOR

How does a physician spend a typical workday? The hours vary somewhat among physician types, but they are usually long. A typical day in my neurology practice starts around 7:00 AM at the hospital making rounds. I grab a cup of coffee and print out a daily census of my patients in the hospital. I make my way to the room where my first patient awaits.

Mary is a seventy-year-old woman who woke up yesterday and fell out of bed. She then realized that her left side was paralyzed and managed to pull the phone off the nightstand to call her daughter. When she tried to talk, her speech was so slurred that her daughter could not make sense of it, so she called an ambulance. Mary has suffered a stroke. She will need a workup for the cause, and treatment for future stroke prevention. She will then need rehabilitation with physical therapy, occupational therapy, and speech therapy in a rehabilitation hospital or nursing home. She can expect a gradual, partial improvement in her deficits, which may take several months. Mary was an active senior citizen before this sudden event. She is worried about who will take care of her dog, her car, her house, and her bills. She begins to cry as I explain that it is doubtful that she will ever be able to return to an independent lifestyle again. After examining her, I review her hospital chart, laboratory results, radiology reports, review her CT and MRI scans, write additional lab and medication orders, and dictate a consultation. I have a frank discussion with her daughter, who must make some plans for her mother's future. It is a difficult situation for the entire family and will change each of their lives in some way. There is nothing I can do to reverse the effects of the stroke at this point, and so my efforts are directed toward identification of risk factors and prevention of another stroke in the future.

The next patient is Bernie, who has Alzheimer's disease. His family brought him to the hospital because they couldn't take care of him at home any more. He has been wandering around the neighborhood and driving his car erratically. He got lost in the local neighborhood twice and was escorted home by the police. He has become incontinent as well, and he is being admitted for nursing home placement. One of the more ridiculous Medicare regulations prevents me from admitting him directly to the nursing home; he can qualify for coverage only if he has a three-day stay in an acute-care hospital prior to transfer to the nursing home.

Bernie becomes very angry with me when I tell him he must give up driving. He vehemently denies that there is anything wrong with his memory. It is well recognized, however, that people with dementia have poor judgment and cause many car accidents. I do not feel guilty about this restriction, although I do feel compassion for this man and his family, who watch his mind slipping away day after day. In some states like California, I would be bound by law to report him to the Department of Motor Vehicles, and they would revoke his license. If I failed to report him in those states, I would be liable for any injury he caused behind the wheel. Even in states without mandatory reporting laws, a good lawyer would find me responsible for any accident he caused if I didn't document that I had instructed him not to drive. Fortunately for other drivers, he won't have access to a car in the nursing home and will soon forget his anger toward me. Sometimes, like a parent, we have to do what in our judgment is best for our patients, even though we may be the "bad guy" in their eyes. Driving is a privilege that can be revoked in people with various health problems like dementia, stroke, and epilepsy. It is typically a physician's responsibility to make decisions about their patient's ability to drive, even though we have very limited time to evaluate them. In addition, we are frequently liable for the behaviors of our patients when they cause harm to others by driving or operating equipment when they have these conditions.

The next patient is Fred, a fifty-eight-year-old alcoholic man admitted through the ER the night before with seizures. It seems that he stopped drinking, and about thirty-six hours later his brain commenced the withdrawal process. He is now seeing bugs on the wall, rambling on about stolen keys to his safe and someone with a gun. As he slips into delirium tremens (DTs), his pulse and blood pressure get dangerously high, he is sweating profusely, and he has a high risk of mortality. As it takes four people to hold him down on the bed, I write orders to sedate him and move him to the ICU for close monitoring and soft restraints. In a few days he'll come back to his senses. He tries desperately to bite and kick me as I attempt to explain why we are tying him down. We frequently see people at their worst, both physically and mentally; it is simply the nature of our work in the medical profession. Sometimes it is hard to maintain a nonjudgmental attitude toward them. Health care workers frequently put themselves at risk when taking care of violent or contagious patients.

After that, I see a thirty-eight year-old woman with a prolonged migraine who is at her wit's end. In between the tears, I find out that there are many emotional issues she is stressed about. Her marriage is unhappy, her teenage children are out of control, and she is anxious about her health as well. Because of my time constraints, I cannot sit with her and listen to all her problems, so I arrange for psychiatric consultation. They will most likely place her on medication for depression and anxiety. As these conditions are treated, her headaches should also improve. People with anxiety disorders and depression usually present to their doctors with various complaints of pain. It is up to the physician to sort out those with physical causes from those with psychological causes of their pain. This can be a very difficult task and often involves running expensive tests to rule out serious medical problems. If the underlying psychological condition is not treated, the patient will often return with persistent symptoms or a new complaint. Often it is easier to give the patient pain medications than to delve into the unresolved issues that lead people to become frequent flyers in the ER or doctor's office. Many times a patient will have severe psychosocial problems with which we cannot help them. There are often issues of abuse, alcohol or chemical addiction, financial problems, or marital strife that may require long-term counseling or lifestyle changes before the physical symptoms improve. However time-consuming, a little reassurance and compassion are often more helpful than a bottle of pills.

I go next to the room of a ninety-year-old woman with osteoporosis, chronic back pain, and pinched nerves. She is very uncomfortable, and there is nothing I can do to reverse the arthritic changes in her back. Surgery would be too risky, but I can assist in pain management. With an adjustment in her medications and physical therapy, I hope to be able to help her reduce the pain and improve her mobility. There are many conditions in which physicians are unable to reverse the changes of aging or disease, so we do what we can to relieve suffering.

Finally, my morning hospital rounds end with the tragic case of a forty-six-year-old man who smoked for twenty years. He was admitted after having a seizure while he was sleeping, witnessed by his wife. His tests show evidence of lung cancer, and it has metastasized to his brain. Today, I must deliver this devastating news to him and his wife, as well as a plan for treatment. I arrange for him to begin radiation and start him on some steroids. I arrange for consultation with a cancer specialist. He will need a biopsy to confirm the diagnosis and to plan treatment. The patient and his wife are clearly trying to comprehend what I am explaining to them, but I can see that I lost them at the word *cancer*. Being the bearer of terrible news is very stressful for physicians too, and, unfortunately, it is a large part of what we have to do on a daily basis. I grab another cup of coffee, take a deep breath, clear my head, and drive over to my office. (Most physicians are addicted to coffee, and I am no exception.)

My first patient in the office is a nineteen-year-old woman who has been having headaches. She has seen my colleague at work, as well as other physicians, for this problem without finding relief. She had been taking so many over-the-counter pain medications that she developed analgesic rebound headaches, which is an increasingly common problem. Her neurological exam was entirely normal, but on her last visit, she said, "My headaches are better, but I'm worried that I may have a brain tumor." When patients say things like that, they usually have anxiety related to their health. However, sometimes they have symptoms they are unable to describe that could be serious. For some reason, a red flag went up in my mind, which may have been a combination of clinical intuition and/or defensive medicine. I ordered an MRI of her brain.

It would have been impossible to get that test approved by her insurance company based on my diagnosis of rebound headaches or on the basis of "intuition." After eleven years in practice, I have learned some tricks of the trade, however, and, with some extra paperwork, the test was done. The people who control the insurance company's managed care decision about various tests are minimally trained; they sit behind a computer with a list of key words or diagnoses that must be given to approve that test. Even the physicians who back them up are often lacking in specialty experience. Physicians usually get savvy about what keywords are needed to get a test approved. People say that most of us doctors are going to hell, since insurance companies have made liars out of us. At least we can justify our lies when our patients get the tests or treatments we feel that they need.

Today my nineteen-year-old comes back so I can tell her that the MRI does indeed show a large brain tumor. Although I don't tell her this at the time, I suspect that the tumor is of a type that may kill her in a matter of months. Her mother, who accompanied my patient to the office, falls apart before my eyes. She can't understand why this tumor wasn't diagnosed earlier by other physicians who treated her daughter. I try in vain to defend them by explaining that her normal neurological exam made a brain tumor very unlikely and difficult to diagnose. The threat of a lawsuit against my colleagues looms in the background as I try to console this young woman and her mother. The brain tumor is unlikely to have been related to the headaches that had actually improved after she stopped the daily pain medications. She still has a normal neurological exam, so the tumor was not producing any obvious symptoms yet. Nevertheless, this family is devastated, and as I refer her to neurosurgery for a brain biopsy and further treatment, I too am devastated and question what good my history and examination were in making this diagnosis. Statistically this patient fell out of the bell curve, but for her it doesn't matter. Young women with headaches are extremely common, and less than 1 percent of them have a serious cause for their symptoms. The most common cause of these headaches is migraine, which affects a large portion of the population and requires treatment but not brain imaging or added tests.

For the rest of the week, this one patient lingers in my thoughts above all others and darkens my mood. I keep reviewing her neurological exam and history to determine whether there were any other clues to the diagnosis. I ask myself why I ordered an MRI on her and not so many others, even though it turned out to be the right decision. However, slow-growing tumors of the brain often push normal tissue out of the way and produce few symptoms until they get very large, making them difficult to diagnose early. We try to detach ourselves emotionally from our patients' problems, but it is nearly impossible to accomplish this all the time. There will always be a few patients with exceptionally good and bad outcomes whom I will remember till I die. I wonder whether any of my patients will remember me years from now.

The next patient is a healthy young male who slipped and fell in a local market and is suing them because there was water on the floor. He is still complaining dramatically, several months later, of severe, stabbing, shooting, knifelike, stinging back pain, but I have found nothing in his X-rays, MRI scans, or nerve testing to explain it. His body language and normal examination contradict his claims. My experience in these situations is that his back pain is unlikely to get better until his liability lawsuit is settled. He brings in several pages of disability and legal forms for me to fill out on his behalf. His lawyer will most likely want me to give a deposition on his behalf, and I don't look forward to it or the cross-examination.

My day continues with an older gentleman with Parkinson's disease who needs a medication adjustment. He is trembling like a leaf and has been very confused recently. The medication he takes makes him dizzy and causes a drop in his blood pressure, yet without these same medications, he is stiff and unable to get out of a chair. We have already tried all the alternative medications, and as he reaches the end stages of Parkinson's disease, I am left with a feeling of impotence in the face of this progressive, incurable disease. His wife, who is about as old and frail as he is has been trying to care for him herself and is having a tough time picking him up each time he falls or gets stuck in a chair. Medicare will not cover home-care assistance and with her children living far away and working, she is in an all-too-common dilemma that the elderly face in this country. If the patient does not improve, his wife will be forced to move him into a nursing home, which Medicare will cover, even though the cost is much higher than home-care assistance would be. I decide to refer him to a movement disorder specialist (a subspecialist in neurology who focuses on Parkinson's disease) at the local university, in the hopes that this colleague will consider brain surgery to help stabilize him for some time. The technology of deep brain stimulation to the parts of the brain responsible for control of involuntary movements has improved a great deal over the past few years and may reverse some of the tremor, allowing the patient to be maintained on a lower dose of medication with fewer side effects. Although the disease will continue to progress, this treatment may help keep him home and more independent for a while.

Next I see a young woman with hysterical complaints of numbness, whose exam does not fit an anatomic pattern of known peripheral nerve or brain disorders. She is terribly depressed, has anxiety and panic attacks, and, as she describes all her symptoms, she cries. She has been to multiple other physicians and has had many tests run, all of which were normal. While I feel sorry for her, I find myself wishing that all my patients had straightforward medical illnesses that I could treat with an objective, unemotional approach. I try as diplomatically as I can to explain that there is no evidence of a physical disorder causing her symptoms, but that her anxiety may be manifesting itself in this way. She does not believe me, and gets very upset, crying even more that there is nothing wrong with her to explain the symptoms. It is very stressful to deal with anxious, depressed patients who are often convinced they have a life-threatening illness, want every test in the book, and have very little insight into the role their psychiatric condition plays in their symptoms. Because we neurologists see so many of these "worried well" patients, it is sometimes difficult to separate the wheat from the chaff and figure out whether there is really any physical basis to the patient's symptoms. We also see patients who have both real medical problems and psychological problems that are intermixed. For example, many patients with epileptic seizures also have pseudoseizures—spells that mimic their seizures but are not brought on by electrical abnormalities of their brains but by stress or anxiety. Treating these patients is very challenging because without continuous monitoring of the brain-wave activity, physicians have to rely on the patient's or family's description of the event. If we increase or add more medication to control epileptic seizures, we run the risk of causing toxic side effects and still not controlling the pseudoseizures. Psychiatric treatments have a poor record for curing patients of the emotional problems that lead to these pseudoseizures, and physicians are often caught in the dilemma of being unable to deal with their patients' emotional baggage successfully.

I recall a patient I once saw while I was in medical school, with a rare psychological condition called Münchausen Syndrome. This young man showed up in the emergency room with complaints of severe abdominal pain and blood in his urine, which was assumed to be caused by a kidney stone. If you have ever experienced one of these kidney stones, you know they can be extremely painful, and high dose narcotics are usually used to treat them in order to make a patient more comfortable while passing a stone. This patient was admitted and given plenty of morphine to make him comfortable. An extensive workup with CT scans of his kidneys and bladder showed no evidence of kidney stones. As the physicians and students on our medical school team scratched our chins, trying to explain the severe pain and blood that had previously been found in his urine, we could find no logical explanation. The attending sent me back into the patient's room to check on his IV solutions, and I caught him trying to poke one end of a coat hanger up his penis into his urethra to cause more bleeding. When I confronted him about it, he denied what I had seen for myself. A psychiatry consultation was ordered, and when the psychiatrist saw the patient, his prognosis for recovery was very guarded. Most patients with Münchausen Syndrome do not improve with conventional psychiatric medications and often become frequent visitors to various emergency rooms, switching to different facilities once they have been identified. When we discharged this patient, he then started listing a host of new complaints. His willingness to harm himself for the sake of proving he had various diseases was confounding, and frustrating for the medical team. What is even worse, however, is a parent who claims various illnesses in his or her child to gain medical treatment for the youngster. This is called Münchausen by Proxy, and I have seen a few of these cases as well. The physical and psychological abuse by a parent with this severe mental illness can do long lasting psychological harm to a child who then becomes convinced that he or she is perpetually sick.

At eleven the pager goes off. The ER has an acute stroke patient I must see immediately if he is going to qualify for TPA. This is a medication that dissolves blood clots and may help reverse the patient's stroke if given within three hours of the onset of his symptoms. There are still two patients in my office, and I go out to the waiting room to explain to them that I will be delayed. One patient gets angry and storms out of the office, and the other decides to wait. I rush to the ER, feeling excited about seeing an emergent patient where I can really make a difference. I arrive in the ER where a sixty-year-old man is lying in a bed, unable to speak or move his right side. He is awake and appears bewildered. His wife anxiously tells me he was eating breakfast with her when he suddenly slumped over, and dropped his fork. The stroke symptoms began one hour ago. A CT of the head shows no bleeding, and his labs are normal. He has no other contraindications, so I explain the potential benefit and the risks of complications, including bleeding and death, that can be caused by TPA. I explain about the time window that exists to preserve brain tissue and the urgency of treatment immediately to open up the blocked blood vessel in the brain. The wife consents to proceed with treatment, since the patient cannot speak for himself, and the infusion is begun. The patient is admitted to the ICU, where he will be monitored closely for the next twenty-four hours. It is exhilarating to be on the front lines of medicine and to feel that what you do can have an immediate impact on your patient's life or death. I suppose that ER physicians and many surgeons get this type of opportunity frequently throughout the day, but as a neurologist, I more often deal in my practice with chronic problems that can be managed but not cured. The treatment of acute stroke has evolved dramatically and has improved the outcomes of our patients with the development of specialized stroke care units in hospitals and rapid treatments to dissolve the blood vessel clots that cause strokes. I was a neurology resident when TPA was being studied, and I participated in the clinical trials that led to its approval by the FDA (Food and Drug Administration) as the first treatment for acute stroke. How gratifying it is now to be able to utilize this treatment with the hopes of reversing the damage being done to this patient's brain. The joy of being able to help another with our hard-earned skills is something that is hard to describe but is what keeps most physicians going, despite the frustrations of medical practice.

I return to the office at twelve thirty to see my last patient of the morning. He is a twenty-nine-year-old chronic pain patient. His symptoms stem from an old neck injury. He brings with him a list of addictive narcotic pain medicines and muscle relaxers he has been getting from another physician, and he wants me to refill them. I try, in my most diplomatic way, to convince him that addictive drugs are not the answer for chronic pain. I give him several suggestions on safer alternative medicines and methods of dealing with the pain, but he ends up storming out of my office, making threats of lawsuits to my staff. We certainly cannot please them all and frequently find ourselves hounded by a few nightmare patients who have us paged at all hours, call the office multiple times per day, and threaten us or our staff if we don't give them what they want. It makes practicing medicine very difficult and stressful at times. Despite the threat of a lawsuit, however, I must be true to the principles of good medicine. This includes prevention of narcotic addiction, which can be much more difficult than simply writing prescriptions for pain medications upon demand.

With the ten minutes left in the lunch hour, I answer some phone messages, drink more coffee, and head back to the hospital to see more patients. My TPA stroke patient is getting better. He can now speak a few words and lift up his right leg. I feel a surge of excitement as I watch him improve, and that helps to relieve the frustration I felt after my earlier patient interaction.

Next I stop in the doctors' lounge, a small room in the hospital where doctors can hide from their patients and their patients' families to eat or relax. Most hospitals have doctors' lounges, where physicians could go to have a cup of free coffee or a free meal, rest a while, catch up on phone calls or test results courtesy of the hospital administration. (These "freebies" are now discouraged as appearing to be a bribe for using the hospital's facilities, and have for the most part been discontinued.) When I first started practice, this was a relatively happy, congenial, and relaxing place to hang out for a few minutes in between patient visits. The conversations in the doctors' lounge used to be upbeat, intellectually stimulating, and light. It was a place to consult colleagues in an informal atmosphere, and regroup before returning to the lives of our patients. You could get a sense of the morale of the medical staff and discuss issues of relevance to the medical community. Lately it seems that complaints about the system, noncompliant and uninsured patients, and the costs of practicing medicine have taken over. Over the years, more conversations have turned to the plight of physicians, especially the difficulties of managing a medical business, liability issues, and general dissatisfaction with the practice of medicine. The morale of physicians these days is very low, and many of my colleagues look for ways to get out of the business of medicine, despite having spent half their lives training for their careers.

After lunch, I return to the office to do some EMGs (nerve tests), read some EEGs (brain-wave tests), dictate notes for all my patients, fill out mountains of forms and papers, and refill prescriptions. I see another eight patients as well. I return some calls from patients with new or worsening symptoms, and, as the day progresses, two more hospital consults come in, so it's back to the hospital for the third time today. Finally I leave the hospital around seven PM and head for home.

Several hours of the day are spent doing paperwork that keep us from our patients and constitute time for which we are not paid. The paperwork mountain has grown considerably over the past several years and now includes phone calls to various insurance companies and managed care companies to justify the need for various tests, treatments, or medications to some person on the other end of the line who has not seen the patient and who lacks the medical knowledge and experience I have regarding the patient's condition.

As I finally walk in the door of my home, the pager goes off again, and it is the ER. There are not many things that can make your heart sink faster than seeing the ER phone number on your pager at night when you are already exhausted. They have a twenty-two-year-old man who has been doing crack cocaine; he has suffered a massive bleed in his brain and is comatose. I apologize to my family, turn around, and rush back to the ER to see this young man. The patient's condition is as bad as it can be, and within a few days, massive swelling of the brain will develop, squeezing his brainstem, where basic life functions are stored, resulting in brain death. His family has arrived, and, as I explain the dismal prognosis for his survival, they cannot accept the situation and simply don't believe me. They demand that I transfer him to another hospital. Since the young man has no insurance, it is difficult to get another hospital to accept him, but eventually we succeed in arranging a transfer to the university hospital. Strokes, hemorrhages, and heart attacks are all-too-common tragedies for young people who never dream that getting high with their friends could lead to these outcomes. Perhaps some good will come from this patient's death if his family agrees to make him an organ donor. Perhaps his friends will realize how dangerous these drugs really are and think twice before smoking crack again.

Finally I am able to return home in time to kiss my children good night. The stress of the patients I saw today is put aside, and I put on the wife-and-mother hat. As I unwind, I pray for a quiet night and wish I could throw my pager in the toilet. Tomorrow I will get up and do it all again.

As a neurologist, I have to spend more time with my patients than most other physicians if I am to be effective. Taking a good, complete history and performing an extensive, detailed exam takes time but can make 80 percent of diagnoses correct. Tests, such as MRIs, EEGs, or EMGs, can be ordered and are usually confirmatory. Most neurological diseases are not curable, but they are treatable. It takes time to educate our patients about their medical conditions and the treatments and medications available. The potential side effects of medications must be explained in detail, and the patient must be assured that you will be there to help him or her deal with what is frequently a chronic condition that may last for years. We often see patients in their older years, when issues centered around independence come up, such as driving or living alone in their own homes. Because we deal with the brain, we see a lot of patients who have coexisting mental illness as well. These issues take time to talk about and must be addressed with the patient for their well-being. It is part of being a good physician to see the patient through their eyes and to help them deal with the practical issues that come up in their daily lives in relation to their medical condition. This is one reason that computers will never be able to replace physicians. The human interaction is important, and, I hope, still appreciated by our patients.

A typical day for a physician can vary quite a bit depending on the type of practice he or she has. I don't presume to know what other types of physicians go through on a daily basis or the stress they have to deal with. I do not experience the joy of performing a successful surgical procedure, or the tremendous anxiety when a patient's condition deteriorates in the operating room under a surgeon's knife. For a surgeon, the day may include some combination of rounds on hospital patients, surgery, patient follow-up and evaluations in the office, and, of course, paperwork. Primary care physicians see many more patients per day in five- to ten-minute appointments, in part due to lower reimbursement for each patient. Pediatricians, who care for the future of our world, are some of the lowest-paid physicians of all. Their days typically include a combination of inpatient and outpatient care and paperwork. What all new physicians find is that several hours of each day are spent not practicing their skills with their patients, but doing paperwork, dictating notes for each patient encounter, filling out forms, and making phone calls. Many patients or their families call their doctors multiple times per day with questions or concerns and seem to think that they are the only patient that the physician has. Messages pile up throughout the day and must be answered. Patients often don't understand why they cannot speak to their physician right away whenever they call. If we were to stop to answer each phone call, the day would never end, and the patients in the office would never be seen. Other physicians call specialists to discuss a case they are evaluating and want a "curbside consult." Pharmacies call in for prescription refills. Laboratories fax over test results or call in critical results that must be dealt with right away. These are understandable interruptions throughout the day, but they can take a lot of time and delay the care that patients waiting in the office receive. It is not uncommon for the ER to call in the middle of the day with a critically ill patient who takes priority over the patients in the office, causing physicians to reschedule those outpatients or keep them waiting, sometimes for hours. Patients in the office often get angry about having to wait, but this is the nature of medicine; the sickest people must be treated first. The end result is that physicians are constantly pulled in too many directions and must prioritize every moment. They may have to rush back and forth between the hospital and the office several times per day, and their workday is not over until everyone has been taken care of, even if the day stretches late into the night.

## THIRTY-SIX-HOUR DAYS, ONE-HUNDRED-HOUR WEEKS

Most physicians work in their offices or hospitals from ten to sixteen hours per day. As you can see, physicians' work hours depend on the number and types of patients they see and are quite unpredictable. When they are on call, they continue working from home. Their pagers can go off at any time throughout a twenty-four-hour period and continue throughout the following work day. They may have to return to the hospital several times for emergent cases. There are also pages from nurses at the hospital, calls from patients or family members at home, prescriptions needing refills or questions that need answering. In fact, the pager can go off twenty or thirty times in a twenty-four-hour period, and fragmented sleep and poor quality family time can result. Then the physician must get up and head back to the office for another full day with little or no rest. A physician's work week typically runs from sixty to one hundred hours or more, depending on how often they are on call.

In solo private practice, the call can last twenty-four hours per day, seven days per week. Single-specialty groups share call coverage, which can be a major advantage. A solo physician cannot leave their practice uncovered when they leave town or take a vacation. They must arrange for another physician to cover their practice in case a patient has an emergency. It is not considered ethical to refer them to the ER, especially when they are specialists. I was on call twenty-four hours per day, seven days per week in my first year of practice. There were a few other neurologists who would cover for me when I went out of town, however. Later in my career, as a private-practice neurologist, I found myself on call for two years straight, without any coverage. I wore the beeper everywhere I went. I was even afraid to miss a page while taking a shower. As a single mother and physician, I found myself juggling my responsibilities to my patients and my children with great difficulty. Each day was a challenge, especially when my kids would get sick or my office schedule ran late, and the kids needed to be picked up at day care. My children spent a lot of time in the doctors' lounge waiting for me to make hospital rounds and eating hospital food. I was the primary caregiver for my mother, who was very ill for a year before she died, and I had to continue making rounds and seeing patients even on the day of her death. It was one of the most difficult times of my life. I barely held back the tears as I took care of my patients, who had no idea of the grief I was trying to suppress. It was all I could do to carry on as if my full attention were on my patients' problems.

When I got remarried, my husband took over most of the domestic duties so that I could work harder and concentrate on my primary responsibility—my patients. For our wedding, I had to hire a locum tenens neurologist to cover for my practice. This temporary coverage for just one week cost me more than the wedding and honeymoon combined.

I used to joke that I wanted a househusband, but in reality, that's exactly what I needed, and while it was difficult supporting a new husband and my own children, I could not have spent the time needed to practice medicine without him, and my children got some much-needed discipline as well. It was especially difficult for the children, since they had to accept this new adoptive father, and I was not around for many of their personal crises and conflicts, but we all dealt with the cards we were given and survived, stronger—I hope—for the experience.

There are very few jobs that are as demanding as medicine, when not showing up to work can literally be a matter of life and death. We are tied to our beepers and expected to be available to our patients anytime, anywhere. We can't leave town, get sick, or have personal excuses for not showing up to work, unless we make arrangements with another physician to cover for us.

We often work so hard that many of us get burned out and lose sight of the reasons we went into medicine, especially when giving our best is not acknowledged, reimbursed or appreciated. The enthusiasm and excitement we started out with is replaced with exhaustion and dread of what crises we will have to face each day. We are dealing daily with sick patients and their anxious families, and strong emotions abound. They often direct their anger, frustration, and fear toward the physicians who are trying to help them. It is difficult to protect ourselves from the stress that is an integral part our lives. The levels of stress experienced by physicians have increased dramatically in the past five to ten years, according to recent surveys, and are at an all-time high (Adams, 2002).

# DEALING WITH INSURANCE
# COMPANIES AND MANAGED CARE

Practicing medicine involves getting various tests and treatments approved by our patients' insurance companies. When hours of our staff's time and written forms fail to get approval, physicians frequently call the insurance company and try to appeal on our patient's behalf. The people who work in these large insurance bureaucracies are frequently not physicians or even nurses and have little or no medical knowledge. Although some managed care organizations have improved their review processes and include more medically trained personnel, it can still be frustrating to spend the extra hours necessary each day to justify testing or medications to someone who has not seen the patient and does not know his or her unique situation as well as the physician who actually saw the patient. We find ourselves having to convince someone in the insurance company what is best for our patients, and if our working diagnosis doesn't contain certain key words, our patients are denied the care we feel they need. Frequently, these companies ask for a diagnosis before they will approve the very test that we need to make the diagnosis. Frequently we find ourselves asking, "If we knew the patient had that diagnosis already, we wouldn't need that test, now, would we?" If we list a diagnosis that a patient does not have but that we are trying to rule out, this goes on his or her insurance records and constitutes insurance fraud. These diagnostic insurance labels can lead to problems for the patient later on when changing insurance (preexisting condition exclusions) and can cause denial of life insurance coverage.

Most graduating residents or fellows join a group or partnership that has an established practice, and over time they learn the ropes. They leave their training excited about practicing the science and the art of medicine but soon find themselves drowning in paperwork that has little to do with patient care. Catering to government regulations, calling insurance companies for approval of tests or treatments their patients need, and filling out endless forms are activities that give them less and less time to care for their patients. When a new patient enters the office, the paper trail has already begun, with the staff getting the referral numbers and information, insurance verification, and authorizations to treat the patient. A chart is made up, and when the patient arrives, they are presented with many forms to fill out and sign, each of which satisfies some regulation by the government or insurance company. At the time of the visit, a two- or three-page history and physical or consultation is dictated and transcribed, and it becomes part of the patient's medical record. This is a narrative of the patient's illness, their symptoms as they describe them, their past medical history, their examination findings, the tests they may have had, and finally, an assessment and plan for further tests and treatments. The reports of their visits and tests are kept in their chart. As thousands of patients are seen over the years, the walls of the office get filled to capacity from floor to ceiling, until boxes of older charts must be culled and placed in storage. These records must be kept for seven years and must be available upon patient request or insurance audit. Prescriptions are written or called into local pharmacies. Tests are ordered by filling out more forms, which require certain diagnoses in order to be covered by insurance companies or Medicare.

A complex electronic bill is generated and must be submitted to the insurance company with perfect accuracy in order to receive payment. Even then, many insurance companies routinely deny payment on a first claim, requiring more documentation and dragging the process on before the physician is finally paid. After the patient leaves, test results come back to the office and are reviewed as they are received. Stacks of laboratory and radiology results are reviewed daily. Patients are notified of the results, and further tests or treatments scheduled as the need arises. Most of the time, the nurse calls the patient or sends a note if she is unable to reach them. The physician may call the patient or the referring physician, depending on the urgency or severity of the situation. Additional tests or referrals to other physicians may need to be arranged. Altogether, there are many hours expended behind the scenes on our patients. As a neurologist, I also insist on reviewing every CT or MRI scan I order, rather than relying on the radiologist's report. Occasionally, knowing the patient and specific location of concern, I find things the radiologist missed. I usually get records from other physicians who have seen the patient, and I review those as well. Patients and their family members call the office throughout the day with concerns and questions about the patients' problems that require time to address. Unlike lawyers, who bill for any time they spend on their clients, physicians can only bill for the time spent directly with the patient in the office, and they must accept whatever payment the insurance company decides to pay. The rest of the time spent on patient care, including phone calls, checking test results, and dictating transcripts of the patient interaction is not reimbursable but takes up several hours of each day.

One of my colleagues was telling me about his frustration with managed care insurance, which would not approve a CT scan of the abdomen for his patient. When the initial written request was denied, he called the insurance company. They put him on hold for ten minutes and then he found himself speaking with a young woman who had no medical training—an office clerk with a computer screen in front of her, listing the only diagnosis codes that would lead to approval of this particular test. Unfortunately those lists are woefully incomplete and don't take into account the myriad factors that can lead great physicians to follow their intuition or think outside the box. This clerk kept asking my friend if his patient had a tumor in the abdomen, and he kept telling her that this was his concern, and the reason he was ordering the test. He was suspicious that she might have a tumor, but he was not psychic, and his physical exam alone was not adequate to rule it out. She had some blood-test abnormalities and abdominal pain, but these were not on the computerized list for approval of the test. After another half an hour of arguing with this young woman, the physician hung up, unable to get the test approved. When he explained this to the patient, her only other option was to pay for the test herself, which she was not willing or able to do. Two months later the patient was found unconscious in her home. She was rushed to the hospital, where she was found to have a ruptured abdominal aneurysm. Unfortunately she passed away, and her family sued my friend for not making the diagnosis earlier and preventing this catastrophe. The managed care organization had placed a legal loophole in the patient's contract to prevent it from being sued in cases where a test was denied. However, the doctor who, months before, went out of his way trying to get the test approved, was found to be liable for the consequences because the lawyers convinced a jury that he hadn't done enough. He became so disillusioned that he retired shortly after that, as have many physicians with experiences like this, which are all too common.

## THE GOOD, THE BAD, AND THE UGLY— PATIENTS AND PHYSICIANS

From a physician's perspective, there are good patients and there are bad patients. We physicians see them all, and we try to treat everyone equally.

However, we are forced into treating people very differently, because of highly variable insurance coverage or lack of insurance. There is definitely a hierarchy of patients, an insurance-driven caste system, and physicians usually end up in the middle of it. It goes against our grain to be forced to provide different levels of care based on the patient's insurance or ability to pay, but we are given no choice by today's system. In addition, individual patient factors such as lifestyle, likelihood of compliance, and liability risk color our medical decision making. This all makes for an incredibly complex combination of factors that physicians must sort through with each patient they see. It is impossible to be perfect in this system, when attempting to consider all of the issues, not just the pure medical ones.

What are good patients? They come in with a good attitude; they want to get well. They are able to give a good history of their present illness, describing their symptoms clearly; if they cannot communicate well, their family members bring them in and help with the history. They can list their other medical problems, and they know what medications they are taking, including dosages. They are honest about their habits like alcohol or smoking, and they cooperate with the examination process. Most important, they are compliant with their physician's recommendations, and take their medications as prescribed. They show up to their appointments on time, and they seem appreciative of the care they receive from their physicians. They are interested in learning about their diseases and accept some responsibility for their illness and the treatment. They have "good" insurance that allows the physician to give them the best tests and treatments available, without interference or denials, even if these treatments are new or expensive. The physician can also be assured that he or she will be paid for the work he or she is doing. Sadly, these good patients are a very small percentage of the patients we see in a given day.

There are also the bad patients. It is important to realize that good people can be bad patients. These people show up at the last minute in crisis—usually in the ER, late at night—having ignored their symptoms for days, weeks, or even months before. They are unable to give a good description of their symptoms; they don't know the names of their medications ("You know, Doc, a little green pill"). They are not honest about their habits ("I only have one drink per day," which happens to be a pint or a fifth) and then when they go into DTs (delirium tremens), we have to figure out what's going on. They are often late for appointments or don't show up, and are noncompliant with their medications.

Some patients are so determined to destroy themselves that it is difficult for a physician to intervene. Dr. Jones, a plastic surgeon, told me about a patient of his who was a real character. He had a propensity for fighting. He even had a restraining order against him from his wife. He ended up in the ER at two AM with a severe facial fracture from a local bar fight. Because this was a displaced fracture, he was taken to the operating room for an open reduction of the fractured bones in his face. When the bone was moved, a severed artery spewed blood over the surgeon, his team, and the operating room. It was very difficult to get control of the bleeding, and the patient required multiple units of blood. After a harrowing several hours of surgery, a successful outcome was obtained, however, and the patient was transferred to the recovery room and then to a hospital room. A few hours later, the surgeon got a frantic call from the nurses, stating that the patient was threatening to commit suicide if he was not allowed to go outside to smoke!

Pain clinics have an especially difficult time keeping a close eye on patients with narcotics-abuse issues. It is very common to these clinics to become clearinghouses for narcotics addicts and pushers, who frequent one or more of these clinics to obtain a free or very cheap supply of drugs every month. Many patients simply want pain pills for themselves, and some sell them to their friends. Then they call the doctor for more pills with excuses like "The dog ate them" or "They were stolen out of the car." Prescription drug abuse has become a major problem across the country. Sometimes physicians even have to play detective and check up on police reports or call local pharmacies to verify our patients' claims. Some patients get multiple prescriptions from different doctors for the same condition. Some steal the whole prescription pad and write their own prescriptions. They show up in the ER having overdosed or having combined the medications with alcohol or drugs and life-threatening illnesses. They often have no insurance and are seen for free, or they have basic coverage that forces the doctor to treat them with fewer tests and less expensive, generic medications that often have more side effects or are less effective. They are also more likely to sue for malpractice when a bad outcome occurs, and they see this as a "get rich quick" scheme.

Some patients forget to bathe or do basic hygiene, and some douse themselves with enough perfume or cologne to knock out an elephant. Some have hidden agendas, like disability or lawsuits that they don't disclose until the end of their visit. A colleague told me about a patient who showed up for her appointment wearing only a fur coat over a negligee. I had a transvestite patient in the hospital once who insisted on wearing bright-red lipstick all the time and his own frilly nightgowns from home. He said, "I wouldn't be caught dead in those droll hospital gowns." Sadly, he had AIDS and did pass away, but he died in style with his dignity and his lipstick on.

One day I was called to perform a neurology consult on a nineteen-year-old girl whose mother had brought her into the emergency room. She had been seen in two other hospital emergency rooms and dismissed as being on drugs or just crazy. Her mother was in tears as she told me that, while her daughter was a little wild, now she could not remember things, her speech was confused, and she had been sleeping excessively for the past several days. The neurological exam revealed that the young woman was indeed encephalopathic, or delirious. Most illicit drug effects should have worn off after a few days, so I made arrangements for her to undergo an MRI of the brain and a spinal tap to determine the nature of her illness. One of the features of the MRI is that it is a huge magnet, and metallic objects must be removed before going into the same room with it. This young lady had pierced eyebrows, tongue, nose, breasts, and yes, even down below. The nurses and her mom had to locate and remove all those piercings before she could undergo the MRI. After the MRI, I rolled her over to perform the spinal tap, and there was the most hideous tattoo in the small of her back of a horned devil with evil eyes surrounded by a pentagram, staring at me. I had to place my spinal needle through the middle of this disturbing tattoo, which was actually pretty interesting. As it turned out, the young woman really was quite ill with a form of encephalitis—an inflammation of the brain usually caused by a virus. Unfortunately, there is no good treatment for this, but it is usually self-limited. Most patients eventually recover, but many never get back to "normal," whether or not you would call her normal before her illness. It is not meant for physicians to judge their patients and treat them differently, but sometimes patients behave in such a way that a serious illness can be missed because the patient's behavior leads even physicians to make false assumptions. It takes a great deal of objectivity to evaluate a patient individually without being fooled by the stereotypes they may present. At the same time, certain lifestyles or habits make a patient statistically more or less likely to have other medical conditions, so physicians have to take into account things like smoking, drug use, sexual persuasion, prior psychiatric problems, etc.

Many of our patients are simply anxious—the so-called "worried well"—and are frequent visitors to the ER or to multiple physicians. They often have vague or inconsistent symptoms that end up costing taxpayers millions of dollars for normal workups. These patients have a bad attitude toward their own health, many have a secondary gain for being sick, like attention from family members, disability payments, workers' compensation, or successful litigation. Being sick is a self-fulfilling prophecy, and there is little the doctor can do to help these people get well. There are many tricks of the trade that help us identify factitious illnesses and symptoms with more of a psychological than a medical basis, but often things are not so clear-cut. People with mental illnesses get sick too, and an underlying medical problem can be missed when it is embellished upon by the dramatic flair exhibited by many of our patients. Physicians often have to make quick judgments about what type of patient they are dealing with as they choose the appropriate tests and treatments. It is not surprising that many of these patients get million-dollar workups for nonexistent illness because of their dramatic symptoms. Physicians are naturally afraid of missing a real underlying medical condition by assuming the patient is simply hysterical or embellishing the severity of his or her pain. Because of the stigma associated with psychiatric disorders and poor insurance coverage for psychiatry, many people never get the help they really need.

What do we do with patients who have dramatic or severe symptoms and no objective evidence of disease? On the one hand, we are our patient's advocate and have a responsibility to help them, even if symptoms are all we have to work with. On the other hand, there are many reasons that a patient may have a secondary gain for being sick. Perhaps they have serious psychiatric problems or are trying to get the attention of other family members. It is very difficult for a physician to sort through these cases and to determine whether their symptoms are due to organic illness or whether they are attributable to an ulterior motive for some secondary gain. While we learn a few tricks to sort out fictitious illness, we cannot measure pain or verify it in any way. A physician's goal for the patient can frequently be at odds with the patient's goal to receive some financial or emotional gain from an illness or accident. Neurologists frequently consult on patients whose symptoms are confusing or inconsistent with known diseases, or whose pain cannot be explained or adequately treated without high doses of narcotics or other scheduled medications. It is the responsibility of the physician to determine whether there is a real underlying illness and avoid giving a patient potentially harmful medications when they are not warranted. The risk of any treatment and even testing must be outweighed by the potential benefit. Patients often expect to receive a prescription or high-level testing. They often expect a referral to a specialist. Many times the experience and knowledge of treating physicians is such that they are able to make an accurate diagnosis without unnecessary tests or referrals to a specialist, and they may determine that no prescription medication is needed.

All patients are human beings and deserve to be treated with compassion and respect. A physician's commitment includes the Hippocratic Oath to help each person to the best of our ability and to do no harm. We end up having to adjust our treatments of patients based on their medical condition, their insurance coverage, the drug formulary and costs, and psychological factors that determine how they will deal with their illness. The choice of a medication or treatment may be influenced by the likelihood that the patient will be more compliant with a medicine that can be taken once per day versus three or four times per day. The likelihood of compliance goes down dramatically with the increase in frequency of the dose of a medicine. It can be extremely complicated to factor in all the issues, medical problems, drug interactions, side effects, allergies, cost, and availability, as well as whether the patient is likely to take the medication as prescribed.

We accept the tremendous responsibility of being physicians when we pick up our diplomas, and most of us try to give 100 percent each day to each patient, but we are only human. Patients must accept some responsibility for their illnesses as well, and be active participants in the healing process. Most diseases are not curable, but they are treatable, even if that treatment involves simply making a terminal patient more comfortable. Most treatments require both our medical knowledge and our compassion—our complete humanity. This is what makes being a physician so challenging.

People can also tell you there are good and bad doctors. Physicians can even tell you they know bad physicians out there who may be incredibly successful. We have talked about the good doctors, but what about the bad doctors? Who are they, and what happened to them that turned them bad?

As physicians learn to cope with the practical aspects of patient care, they sometimes lose sight of the ideals with which they started their careers. The frustrations of dealing with difficult patients, insurance companies with managed care, business losses, and the long hours demanded of them can cause good physicians to go bad. The motivation to make more money can make good businessmen, but is bad for physicians. The field of medicine is like no other business, as the primary goal cannot be to make money. Yet, in lieu of the spiritual and emotional rewards of patient care, which are dwindling rapidly, many physicians substitute monetary rewards, and many have come to prefer a business approach to their careers. They see themselves as technicians rather than healers. The pharmaceutical industry, the insurance industry, and even hospitals and health care facilities all have profit as the main reason for their existence. Physicians, however, are held to a higher standard. Physicians are expected to deliver patient care to all, regardless of whether they get paid or how much they get paid, which is determined by insurance companies and the government.

Many physicians have found ways to supplement their incomes by buying into radiology testing facilities, laboratories, or outpatient treatment or surgery centers. This in itself may not seem like a bad thing, but when a physician sees a patient with back pain, for example, and refers the patient to get an MRI in which he has an ownership stake, there is a conflict of interest that may lead to unnecessary testing in order to make money. Is this a significant problem? Several studies have determined that self-referral of imaging tests like CT, MRI, and nuclear cardiac scanning is a huge problem (Kilani et al., 2011). It is one of the reasons the cost of health care has risen so much in the last several years.

There are those who succumb to using the drugs they prescribe for recreational purposes or to self-medicate for depression or other problems. Their judgment becomes clouded, and they cannot perform their duties well. The saying, "The doctor who treats himself has a fool for a patient" is very true. Yet the risk of having a psychological problem or substance abuse on your record can affect your ability to get licensed or hospital privileges. There are those who latch on to the latest gimmick to make an extra buck, whether or not it is medically necessary. There is the surgeon whose hands are less skilled, the internist who cannot remember all the diagnoses or treatments involved in a particular case, the lazy physician who finds excuses not to come in to the ER to see a patient in need. There are those who would rather write a prescription for narcotics and keep their patients drugged up, rather than finding the underlying cause of their problems and treat that. There are even a few physicians out there who intentionally do harm to their patients through physical, emotional, or sexual abuse.

Even a great physician can have a bad day or an individual encounter with a patient that goes poorly. They may simply be overtired or have some personal stressors they are dealing with. They may lose their patience with all the demands placed on them and give less than 100 percent effort. They may take out their frustration on their staff, hospital employees, their fellow colleagues, or their patients. When they go home, their families may also bear the brunt of their anger.

## REMEMBERING "THE GOOD OLD DAYS"

Most middle-aged and older physicians wish for the old days, when practicing medicine was very different. There was respect for physicians and no interference with their diagnostic workups or treatment choices. They did what they felt was right for their patients, without insurance companies or Medicare denying the tests or treatments they ordered. People recognized that the field of medicine contains many unknowns, and cures were not always possible. When a bad outcome occurred, the physician could say, "I did everything I could," and families could accept that and go on. People understood that their physician was unable to cure or even diagnose some of their problems. They knew that their doctor had tried his or her best, and that was good enough. Their first thought was not always a potential lawsuit and the riches they could obtain from a bad outcome.

The doctor was like a member of the family, and they had long-term relationships with their patients that allowed for an intimate relationship to grow. Doctors were an important part of their communities as respected leaders and friends. There was a sacred trust between patient and physician that developed after years of knowing each other. Patients appreciated their doctors, thought of them during the holidays, and the doctor-patient relationship could span generations. There was a bond of trust, compassion, and intimacy with the family physician that was sacred and fulfilling to both patient and physician. Now, people change physicians so frequently that these intimate, mutually rewarding relationships rarely have time to develop between doctor and patient.

Insurance reimbursement in the past was high enough to allow doctors to take their time with patients, to absorb the costs of seeing uninsured patients, and really delve into the whole person they were treating, not just a single symptom or an organ system. The time physicians have to spend with each patient has been whittled down so much that there is no time to ask how Mr. Jones's crops are doing, or to hear about the newest grandchild in the family. The regulation of medical care by managed care and the government is not selecting the best physicians but those who can see the most patients in the least time and order the fewest tests and treatments.

Physicians over fifty are retiring early in huge numbers because of the problems with managed care and malpractice as well as the loss of the spiritual rewards that were once an integral part of the doctor-patient relationship (Merritt, Hawkins and Associates, 2000; Merritt, Hawkins and Associates, 2004). They cannot accept the changes that have been forced upon us by insurance companies and the government, and the change in attitude toward physicians that has dehumanized the doctor-patient relationship. Something important has been lost in today's fast-paced, stressful world of medicine, something physicians and patients need to salvage in order to prevent the physician shortage crisis that is imminent in medicine today.

# CHAPTER 3:
## THE BUSINESS OF MEDICINE

Doctors deserve to make a good living after they sacrifice half of their lives to train and endure countless sleepless nights providing care for the sick, don't they? Are doctors any less deserving than sports heroes or movie stars, who make ten to twenty times what most physicians make? Why does it seem that most people think doctors make too much money? Are the challenging and expensive education, hard work and intelligence required to be a physician not supposed to be rewarded in our society?

Where are our priorities as Americans when it comes to having equal access to health care? Don't most people believe that everyone should have medical coverage with the highest level of quality, regardless of their station in life? Why don't our laws and government structure reflect those beliefs?

These days many physicians feel as though they are taken for granted. They are expected to be available for everyone at all times. They are expected to deliver perfect medical care to everyone at all times, regardless of their patients' ability to pay for it. They are almost never paid what they charge for their services. Physicians are placed in a different category from all other businessmen. Their hands are tied when it comes to controlling their overhead or their incomes. They are continually pulled into moral and ethical conflicts over being good physicians and being good businessmen.

## HUMBLE BEGINNINGS

When I started out in 1992, I had finally completed my neurology training and was ready to take on the world. I inherited a private practice from a neurologist in San Diego who was leaving the area. I had looked at several other jobs, from working with other physicians in single-specialty groups, to hospital-sponsored positions, to employment with large, managed care, multispecialty groups. I thought, *What an opportunity, to hang out my own shingle and work for myself!* "Just sign these insurance forms, lease agreements, and hospital privilege applications," this neurologist said, "hire yourself an office manager to do your billing, and you will be a provider. It's easy. The other doctors will start sending you patients, and you'll do fine." I signed every contract that came across my desk without reading them thoroughly or having a lawyer review them, and sure enough, I got busy seeing patients very quickly. I had no money to pay a lawyer to review these contracts I could make no sense of myself. I was in naive trust mode, and it felt great! It was such an exciting time for me; finally, at the age of thirty-five, I was able to call myself a neurologist and begin my career. Unfortunately, the money for services rendered was not as forthcoming as the patients were. There was the managed care company who sent me a notice that they were unable to pay my bill due to financial difficulties, and that they would be paying only 50 percent of their "adjusted charges" over ten years. This amounted to about 25 percent of my usual fees. They went under, but not before the CEO got away with a three-million-dollar bonus. The physicians in the HMO never did get fully reimbursed. I lost over $50,000 on that fiasco. Then there was the patient I saw with carpal tunnel syndrome. First she saw her primary physician, and it had taken a month to get a referral and an appointment to see me, a neurologist. Then it took another three weeks to get approval for her nerve conduction test to confirm the diagnosis and the severity of her condition and another three weeks to get approval for a surgical referral. It took another month to get an appointment with the only hand surgeon on the provider list. It was another month before she finally got the carpal tunnel surgery she needed. Four and a half months to get a relatively simple problem taken care of! Exaggeration? I'm afraid not.

Delays in obtaining care is a common criticism of national health care systems, like the one in Canada but is just as big a problem in America under managed care. The delays in care for many patients in HMOs were longer and filled with more paperwork and wasted time. Compared to HMOs, the physicians' motives are to treat patients and take the best possible care of them. We are rewarded, not punished, for the amount and quality of the work we do.

Many physicians in California and elsewhere were being forced to accept "capitated" payment plans by managed care insurance companies. These plans pay a physician or group a fixed amount of money per enrollee per month in the insurance plan. The physicians were expected to provide all necessary care to the patients referred to them from that plan, regardless of the number or the severity of their illnesses, and regardless of the number of procedures or surgeries they might need. This practice essentially transferred all the risk from the insurance companies onto the backs of the physicians. Physicians who were unwilling to accept these terms were simply shut out, and patients were transferred to their competition. In San Diego there were two excellent groups of ophthalmologists in my region, and they were each presented with a capitated managed care contract. They would be paid a fixed amount and expected to care for all of the ophthalmologic problems that arose among their enrollees. One group accepted the capitated plan, and the other declined. Both groups suffered. The group that refused to sign the capitated contract was driven out of town for lack of patients. The other group was so busy with managed care patients that they lost money on their contract for the hours they spent. There was a six- to twelve-month waiting list for cataract surgery for the patients on this plan.

One day I was called by a local internist. He asked me to consult on a patient of his who was on her way to the ER. She was a nineteen-year-old who had developed numbness from the waist down. When I saw the young woman, I determined that she had transverse myelitis—inflammation of the spinal cord—and would need to be admitted. I called her internist, but he refused to admit her or even follow her while she was in the hospital. He explained that he only got a fixed amount for each enrollee in that plan, and that he would lose money, since he was not going to be paid any extra for coming to the hospital to see this patient. Of course, I admitted the patient and took care of her, but it shocked me, as an idealistic young physician, that other physicians were allowing financial concerns interfere with their medical and ethical decision-making processes. Under these plans, the less a physician does for their patients, the more profit they make. The physicians who are providers for these capitated plans quickly get overwhelmed with patients. The insurance companies, through capitation plans, have successfully shifted the risk to their providers, while continuing to collect the health insurance premium with a set and guaranteed profit.

As in the case of the ophthalmologists, the value of medical care delivered exceeded the amount of fixed reimbursement they received each month. If just a few patients became critically ill, the additional amounts of time spent caring for them would result in a loss of income and ultimately the physicians' jobs. They were motivated to provide as little care as possible to make a profit, just as the insurance companies were. It was not uncommon for patients to wait four to six months for elective surgeries or other nonemergency care.

Some of the Medicaid HMOs I had joined up with denied payment for services I rendered because they determined, in retrospect, that the two AM ER neurology consult I performed was not necessary. Others went out of business after they collected the prepaid fees from the state and federal government for patient enrollment. Of course, they dissolved these businesses before their physicians' charges and hospital bills were paid. Medicaid patients were transferred from one managed care organization to another, and no one took any financial responsibility for the bills that the previous company had accrued. There were denials for payment for various tests I performed because the final diagnosis didn't match the approved list of diagnoses for that test, even though the tests were necessary to rule out those diagnoses. I had to learn the "key words" to use to get tests approved, and how to manipulate the system to play the insurance companies' games. It wasn't a matter of practicing good medicine; it was a matter of documentation in such a way as to get paid or to get approval for a test or treatment. They certainly didn't teach me these things in medical school. I ended up moving away from California to get away from managed care, which had become unbearable for me as a solo private-practice physician.

The first few years of private practice were a tremendous learning experience. The reality of medicine as a business became clear to me, and it was a rude awakening. However, I was dedicated to making my new career a success. Although I billed over $400,000 in charges, my collections were approximately half of that, and the overhead took half of the collections, while taxes and insurance costs took up another 40 percent of what was left. This formula, when carried out, means that from the $400,000 dollars' worth of work in charges, I actually got to keep about 20 percent. Since I could not declare a loss for services rendered that were not reimbursed, the uncollected accounts receivables began to accumulate into the hundreds of thousands of dollars. Unlike many businesses that write off their losses from unpaid bills, physicians have no such tax breaks, and their taxes are very high. I moved to Tennessee to work with a friend who had been a resident with me in California. I worked for her for two years, and on the last day of my employment contract, she fired me, admitting that she simply didn't want to make me a partner. She hired another six or seven different neurologists over the years, each lasting about two years, and never attaining partnership status. I then worked in solo private practice, on call 24/7, having to pay a locum tenens neurologist to cover for even a weekend off. Since then I have worked in small and large group practices, as a locum tenens physician and as assistant professor in a large university practice. I found that certain basic issues prevail in all of these practice models, and they are troubling for all physicians. The individual physician can delegate the business dealings to administrators in large groups, but they give up control over their business, and they relinquish their autonomy. I, like so many other physicians, felt a rising dissatisfaction with the business side of practicing medicine.

## THE COSTS OF PRIVATE PRACTICE

Running a business is difficult for anyone, but owning and operating a medical practice has become so complex and expensive that few physicians are willing or able to manage it anymore. There are so many government regulations that are incredibly strict, and the penalty for a single mistake can run in the tens of thousands of dollars. The overhead costs of maintaining an office have been rising steadily. Malpractice insurance rates have skyrocketed, contributing to a large percentage of the cost increases. At the same time, it's a joke to talk about what doctors charge. Doctors almost never receive what they charge for their services. The amount we are paid for services rendered is determined by the patients' insurance companies, Medicaid, or Medicare. Every time Medicare cuts their reimbursement rates to physicians, the insurance companies follow suit. These rates have been declining steadily over several years. Physicians in private practice have adjusted to these lower payments for their services over the past ten years, but now they are reaching the critical point where they are being forced to close their doors. Medicine is being taken over by big businesses that run physician practices with the emphasis on quantity, not quality. Physicians are pressured by managed care and decreasing reimbursements to see more and more patients in less and less time, in order to make ends meet. Anyone who has been to a physician lately can appreciate the time constraints that physicians are under, as they may get only five or ten minutes with their doctor to explain their symptoms, be examined, and receive treatment. With the increasing use of nurse practitioners and physician assistants, they may not see their doctor at all.

Everyone knows that the cost of health care, from insurance to prescription medications to hospitalization has skyrocketed. If the costs of health care have gone up so much, and physician reimbursements have gone down, where is all the money going? One doesn't need to look far. Pharmaceutical companies, insurance companies, managed care companies, and the legal system have some questions to answer for the American public. These companies depend on physicians and patients for their livelihood, yet physicians and their patients are allowing these companies to remain in control of our health care dollars. The middlemen have taken control of both ends of the financial equation. Patients and physicians are paying the price while these companies reap huge profits.

# PHARMACEUTICAL COMPANIES AND HEALTH CARE COSTS

Pharmaceutical companies in America are an integral part of health care. The major developments in treating disease have been due to the research and production of medications and devices. For physicians, these are the common tools we use to treat our patients. Physicians and pharmaceutical companies work hand in hand to develop new drugs or devices. Physicians in universities across the country help pharmaceutical companies test their new drugs in clinical trials, and these companies get a patent on any new medication that is developed for a specific medical use. In theory, this helps the pharmaceutical company recoup the expense of research and drug development. Their charges are not controlled or regulated like physicians' charges, however, and if you know someone who needs a fairly new brand-name medication, you know that the prices have become astronomical. Without prescription benefits they are simply unaffordable for most people. A drug patent is supposed to expire twenty years after the initial filing patent of a chemical that appears promising in the lab, but it may take ten or more years for the drug to be approved and marketed. There are also many exceptions that can extend this patent, such as approval for a new use of an established medicine, and the time it takes for additional testing required by the FDA. Once the patent expires, cheaper generic drugs can be produced and compete for the prescription dollars, saving Americans millions of dollars. Lately, however, many drugs that should have gone off patent years ago are still not available for generic production because of loopholes in the patent laws. These pharmaceutical companies initiate long and tedious lawsuits that tie the hands of the generic pharmaceutical companies, allowing for bigger profits for the initial developers of a successful drug. That means millions of dollars for each day the competition is held at bay, so what's a few hundred thousand for the lawyers? It's all about big business.

Neurontin is a very popular medication developed originally for epilepsy. It has been on the market since it was initially approved by the FDA in 1994. The generic name is gabapentin, and the patent expired in 2004. Generic versions of gabapentin were developed and marketed at much lower cost to the public. Brand-name Neurontin is very expensive. Because the drug was approved for the treatment of pain several years later, the FDA granted Pfizer, the pharmaceutical company that makes Neurontin, an extension on the patent until 2017. Lawsuits against the generic manufacturers were ultimately successful in forcing these companies to stop manufacturing the generic drug and pay fines to Pfizer for patent infringement.

Physicians around the country have been using Neurontin for nerve pain for years since its emergence on the market. Needless to say, the price of Neurontin has not gone down in all this time but has increased. The pharmaceutical representatives have been marketing it as some sort of panacea, good for whatever ails you, and Neurontin became a best-selling drug for Pfizer, with billions of dollars in sales. Side effects were significantly downplayed in presentations, in fact it was portrayed as being safer than most other drugs in its class. It was also used extensively as a treatment for the mentally ill. However, an increased risk of suicide was found to have been known and covered up, for which Pfizer was sued. Pfizer was eventually found out, and paid $141 million in fines in 2009. A drop in the bucket for them, compared to their profits. Warner Lambert, the company that originally made Neurontin was fined $430 million for off-label marketing In 2004. (Wikipedia.org) It appears that these greedy corporations whose primary motive is profit will never learn about human values, survival, peaceful and natural living, and the Golden Rule. Corporations, through their control over our government may influence the laws the rest of us must live by, but occasionally one gets their hand caught in the cookie jar.

The pharmaceutical companies are in business to make money. However, they need to be controlled either by being held accountable for their prices or by consumers simply refusing to buy their products. It must be made easier for the generic pharmaceutical companies to take over production after the profits reach a certain level, or after a fixed amount of time, without exceptions. Boycotting a drug that may benefit a patient is ethically wrong, but so is accepting the price gouging going on in the pharmaceutical industry. They need to shoulder a portion of the health care burden we all struggle each day to pay. In the past several years, prices for the most commonly used drugs have been rising by double-digit percentage rates every year (Beasley et al., 2011).The only explanation for these increases has been that the overall volume of sales has gone down, so prices were propped up to maintain corporate profits. Some patents are going to expire, and there is a dearth of new products in the pipeline, which has raised concerns about the future profits for the top pharmaceutical companies. In addition, the pharmaceutical companies blame the new health care reform law that was enacted in March 2010, which includes an excise tax on these pharmaceuticals in the future. Bargaining power with the pharmaceutical companies was intentionally limited in the Medicare Part D legislation that was passed under President Bush's term. Why? To appease the industry that has some of the biggest lobbying efforts in Washington. With their income guarantees and legal loopholes they pay little or no taxes and enjoy record growing profits while the rest of the country suffers. Even the middle income, working Americans with pension plans are seeing their 401k's on a rollercoaster ride to nowhere while CEOs earn five to fifteen billion dollar salaries. I say, "People Before Profits!"

More recently drug shortages have become a major issue in the United States. These are blamed on "production issues" by the pharmaceutical companies. Imagine how an oncologist explains to his patient with leukemia that the life-saving, curative drug needed to treat his cancer is unavailable. Where are the ethics in this situation?

Essential cancer drugs have been hit the hardest, but drugs for heart patients, some antibiotics, and intravenous drugs have also been hard for hospitals to find. Hospitals have reported the worst shortage in nearly a decade of chemotherapy agents like doxorubicin. In other words, some of the life-saving, although less expensive, cancer drugs cost more to manufacture, so the drug companies simply stopped or reduced their production in favor of newer, more expensive drugs. In 2010, there were 211 drugs in short supply and almost 300 drugs for 2011. Since profit is the key motive, and no regulatory controls existed with regard to drug shortages, pharmaceutical companies could pick and choose to discontinue manufacture of a three-dollar generic drug that can cure cancer, in favor of a $90,000-drug that can only extend life for a few months (Nelson, 2011). As of October 31st, 2011, President Obama signed an executive order instructing the FDA to take a more active role in reporting of potential drug shortages, expedite regulatory reviews that can help prevent shortages, and examine whether potential shortages have led to price gouging (Salahi, 2011).While this may not go far enough to prevent price gouging, it is at least a step in the right direction.

Under our current system, complex formularies for each insurance plan define what the plan considers acceptable treatment for a variety of illnesses and what they will pay for. There is no regard for the individual decision-making process that goes into the physician's choice of the best medication for their individual patient. The medications that make the preferred list are the least expensive for the insurance company, but not necessarily the best for the patients. Physicians have to keep all this information in mind each time they see a patient, comparing it to what the ideal treatment would be. If insurance isn't going to cover a particular medication, there is no point in mentioning it to the patient. This raises the hopes of a patient anxious to get well and then dashes that hope because the insurance company won't pay for the medication the physician has determined is best. Sometimes there is no effective and safe alternative, and the patient must settle for a drug with more side effects or do without. Patients rarely choose or can afford to pay for the medication themselves. At the same time, if the cost of the drug is outrageously high, and a generic is available, why make the insurance company and the patient pay for the high-priced brand-name medication? The physician is forced to be the middleman between the pharmaceuticals and insurance companies and our patients.

Pharmaceutical companies spend an excessive amount of money and effort developing drugs that are essentially equivalent to a product that a competitor has had success with. They are all building mousetraps, each one competing to make them a little better. We as physicians are barraged with multiple new drugs in the same class and with equal efficacy by aggressive pharmaceutical marketing teams. Expensive TV advertisements proclaim the benefits of their brand, hoping that patients will go to their doctors demanding a medicine they saw on TV. It is cheaper for drug companies to produce a "me-too" drug, than to come up with a novel drug with new characteristics or benefits in treating diseases that don't already have effective treatments. However, the prices of these "me-too" drugs are just as high or even higher than that of the original drug in a particular class.

For example, Imitrex is a brand-name medication for migraine, which was the first in its class and became available around 1991. It is manufactured by Glaxo Smith Kline. I was fortunate enough to take part in the clinical studies on this medicine during my residency. The medication, whose generic name is Sumatriptan, could only be given as an injection at the time. We enrolled in the studies a large group of migraine sufferers who had frequent, severe headaches with no relief from over-the-counter medications. It was a double blind placebo controlled study, which means that neither the doctors nor the patients knew whether they were getting the active drug or a placebo injection.

I remember a young woman who frequented the ER at least once a month and took high doses of narcotics and caffeine, sedatives—anything she could get her hands on to take the edge off these migraines, and when she had one, all you had to do was to look at her face to tell that she was in severe pain. She had enrolled in the study on Imitrex, and when her typical migraine hit, she dragged herself into the office. Bloodshot eyes, pale and pitiful, she lay on the exam table, her eyes covered up with her jacket, lights turned off. In rushed the medical team, which was composed of about four of us med students, as well as residents and the neurology attending physician. With a carefully labeled syringe filled with what, we did not know—either a saline placebo or the active drug—and a quick jab in the arm, and it was done. While we monitored our patient's vital signs, we were witnesses to a most remarkable transformation. Within a few minutes, she began to feel warm all over and described a rush-like sensation in her head. She described a tingling feeling that spread like a wave from the front of her head to the back. This lasted a few more minutes, and as it gradually receded, the headache and, along with it, the nausea, and the light and sound sensitivity all began to improve. Her color improved, her eyes brightened—all within a half hour. Soon she was literally bouncing out the door, stating she had things to do that day—shopping, playing, ready to get her life back on track. It was nothing short of a miracle to watch the effects of this amazing new medication. This new drug really worked, and it was pretty obvious that this was no placebo. There was a new, effective, non-narcotic treatment for migraine, a disabling, if not life-threatening, condition.

Over the next several years we were barraged with a whole host of new migraine medications, each with slightly different chemical structures, but whose effects in binding to certain receptors in the brain were similar. They had slightly different side-effect profiles, and some had better efficacy than others, but overall, the world would have been just as well off without six medicines that basically did the same thing with only a slight molecular difference. The focus of the pharmaceutical industry has gotten off track, and cures for cancer, heart disease, Parkinson's and Alzheimer's diseases and diabetes have not been sought fully enough. It's a waste of valuable resources in favor of grabbing a piece of the "migraine" pie or the quick and easy health care dollar.

There has been much publicity recently regarding the way pharmaceutical companies charge Americans much higher prices for the same drugs than they do patients in other countries. Many people are going across the borders or working with physicians or pharmacies in Canada, Mexico, or Europe to get access to medications that are on average 30 to 50 percent cheaper than they are in the United States. The pharmaceutical lobbyists succeeded— with the FDA's help—in getting legislation passed that restricts Americans from buying their medications from foreign pharmacies. Why aren't Americans outraged that pharmaceutical companies get away with this? Why don't we put a stop to it? These powerful pharmaceutical corporations and their lobbyists justify this in the name of drug development costs. They claim that other countries cannot afford to pay the same prices as Americans for their medications. Can we Americans afford to absorb the costs of drug development alone? Can we afford to increase profits for the pharmaceutical companies while our senior citizens choose between medicine and food? Should those people without prescription drug benefits pay higher prices when across the border, the same medication is available at a fraction of the cost? If we as a country can pass fair-trade agreements that take labor across our borders, why can't we benefit from fair trade for medications made in America, at lower prices? The FDA needs to support legislation that works for the people, not for the pharmaceutical companies.

There is another issue in medicine that physicians and patients must deal with daily. It is the controversy between alternative medicine and traditional allopathic medicine. In medical school I was instructed to forget all that "hogwash" that was based on anecdote or empiric trials, rather than double-blind, placebo-controlled trials. Practitioners of alternative medical treatments were dismissed by the medical profession summarily as quacks or snake oil salesmen. The "body work" I did prior to medical school was laughed at, and the idea of energy fields around people or auras that could be seen and altered by some practitioners was considered preposterous. (The existence of an aura or energy field surrounding people has been shown by new imaging techniques, although its significance is still controversial in allopathic medicine.) However, there are many benefits to alternative medicine that are complementary to benefits of traditional medicine. I think that we may be throwing the baby out with the bathwater when we disregard the beneficial effects of many herbs, nutrition, healing, chiropractic care, and acupuncture. Perhaps we have become so institutionalized and science-oriented in medicine that we forget how little we know, and, in our arrogance, we discount the things we don't understand. Naturally occurring substances often have unrecognized and unproven benefits. Many pharmaceuticals are derived from medicinal plants. Chiropractic treatment, massage, and acupuncture often help release the body's own healing mechanisms. These "touching" specialties offer people something traditional medicine forgets in our objective, alcohol-swabbed world. I try to incorporate some of these alternatives into my traditional practice, even though they may be somewhat controversial. I touch my patients and let them feel my compassion and concern. But then I've always been a hugger. I may recommend a balanced approach that includes herbs and nutritional supplements, chiropractic treatments, or acupuncture in addition to the traditional allopathic treatments. Sometimes I find myself subconsciously channeling energy to them. However, many physicians are afraid of the risks involved in recommending anything that they haven't been exposed to in medical school, or that has not been thoroughly tested in double-blind, placebo-controlled studies which are impossible to effectively design for many of these modalities.

Many of the alternative approaches to health care such as herbs and vitamins have not been studied well enough for medical science to call them safe or effective. There have been examples of herbal supplements that have been shown to be harmful over the years. Tryptophan was used widely in the eighties as a sleep remedy. It was found to cause a serious inflammatory muscle disease—I wrote a paper about this while I was in neurology residency—and was eventually removed from the health food shelves. Megavitamin kicks have led to overdoses of certain vitamins. There have been many other complications of alternative treatments. In order to study the safety and effectiveness of a treatment for disease, rigorous clinical trials are needed. However, to perform the double-blind studies needed to prove a benefit would take a lot of money that no one but the pharmaceutical companies is willing to pay. The pharmaceutical companies sponsor the majority of medical research in this country now. If there is no chance of a profitable prescription drug for the pharmaceutical companies to market, there is no incentive for these companies to support the research. Government funding has been cut back and spread out over so many fields that it is very difficult to support research on public funding alone. Avoiding research on herbs and nutritional supplements is not always in the people's best interest, however. The people need more inexpensive methods of disease prevention and treatment. But it is in the financial interests of the pharmaceutical companies to keep alternative medicine and treatments out of the marketplace.

Pharmaceutical companies used to educate and encourage physicians to prescribe their drugs with various perks, like trips to exotic locations, free golf or tennis trips, or fancy dinners out with paid specialists promoting their drugs. They were wined and dined, along with their spouses, which made for a pleasant night out with colleagues. The pharmaceutical salesmen's attempts to influence physicians to prescribe their drugs were not too subtle, but at least physicians were trained to analyze the data presented and make an educated decision as to whether the drug was appropriate for their patients. Critical analysis of experimental studies is an integral part of medical education, so most physicians take the pharmaceutical advertising and incentives with a grain of salt. Some pharmaceutical companies, however, are more heavy-handed and influence academic research through funding and by altering manuscripts prior to publication. Under threats of government sanctions, the pharmaceutical companies have "self-regulated" some of these incentives.

Physicians, after working hard all day, used to look forward to a free night out at a good restaurant with their spouses and the camaraderie of their colleagues. It was one of the few medically related perks a doctor could look forward to. These meetings allowed physicians to interact with their local colleagues as well as experts and discuss how certain diseases are managed, gaining from their experience with new medications. We are well enough educated to recognize the sales pitches for what they are and to analyze the actual data to make our own conclusions. Now, physicians are expected to attend educational programs after hours—without our spouses, who are already feeling neglected. The extra cost of including our spouses is insignificant when considering the overall marketing dollars these pharmaceutical companies spend. There is a benefit for the spouse attending one of these functions, even if they don't understand the science. It helps them to appreciate the importance of the work that keeps their spouses away so much. After all, the spouse's sacrifice and support in a medical family should not be underestimated.

Now billions of marketing dollars are directed toward medically naive patients, through television and magazine advertisements. If physicians are thought to be too impressionable to sort out the clinically relevant information from the pharmaceutical sales reps, then what about the general public, which is now being barraged with television, magazine, Internet, and radio advertisements? Who knew that male erectile dysfunction was so important that men needed to be ready twenty-four hours a day with a choice of several Viagra-like drugs? The millions of dollars spent on television ads could be funneled into cancer research or production of those medications that are in short supply. What we need is more research on novel drugs for the difficult diseases. Physicians need better tools to work with in order to be effective, and to have more say in what research gets funded.

Spending on prescription drugs in the United States reached $141 billion in 2001. This was the third-largest component of the health care dollar, and it had grown 40 percent since 1990. In 2005 spending on prescription drugs grew to $252 billion. In 2007 the cost had increased to $287 billion (Hoffman et al., 2009). It has continued to rise ever since then at frightening rates. The top ten pharmaceutical companies comprise about 60 percent of the prescription drug market. These companies have powerful lobbyists and tremendous influence on the government. They are motivated to increase their profits, and while their contributions to medical science cannot be denied, remember that they are businessmen first. Anyone that keeps track of the stock market knows that pharmaceuticals are among the most profitable companies in America today. The wealthy invest in these companies to assure themselves of consistent profits. The multimillion-dollar salaries of the CEOs of these companies are coming out of each of our pockets, with every prescription we fill. Mergers are creating a handful of powerful corporations at the top that control the market by the almighty dollar. While the cost of medications has risen exponentially, pharmaceutical companies have successfully lobbied to keep Medicare and other insurance companies from negotiating significant price controls and to deny individuals the right to obtain these same medications from other countries at lower prices. The pharmaceutical companies spend tens of millions of dollars each year in lobbying congress and for campaign contributions. From 1998 to 2006, this industry spent $855 million on lobbying (Ismail, 2005). It is no surprise that the beneficiaries of this money voted as they did on bills affecting drug prices and controls, as well as importation (Dilanian, 2007). They exert control over our politicians to benefit from tax loopholes, to prevent capitalism from applying to their businesses, and by preventing their biggest customer, Medicare from bargaining for lower prices. In recent years, more and more pharmaceutical companies are even outsourcing their research and development to developing countries like India, while cutting jobs here in America (Mercer, 2009).

The new Medicare part D prescription benefit certainly provides some benefits to seniors by covering more of their medications, but it is flawed by a restriction against negotiating prices with the pharmaceutical companies. This additional coverage is raising the cost of health care for all of us and putting that money into corporations that are not even using that money to save jobs here at home. At a time when physicians and hospitals accept a huge, government-imposed reduction on their fees, why aren't the pharmaceutical companies expected to accept the same? The patient is the one who pays, with higher prescription prices and insurance rates.

The physician's hands are tied when a sick patient cannot afford to get a necessary treatment for financial reasons. This is extremely stressful for physicians, as well as patients and their families, and can mean the difference between life and death. I had a young patient with multiple sclerosis, or MS, who came to see me with some numbness and tingling of her left side. Initially, she thought she had slept wrong, but as the day progressed, the symptoms did not go away. She eventually went to the ER, and I was consulted for a neurology evaluation. Upon further questioning, she admitted to having had other odd symptoms that would come and go over days or weeks during the past six months. On examination, she had some abnormalities that heightened my suspicion, and with the results of an MRI of the brain, it became clear to me that MS was the most likely diagnosis. I sat down with her and explained what was wrong, how this disease is incurable, but that new treatments with which she would learn to inject herself could help prevent flare-ups or exacerbations of the disease and could help prevent or delay disability. I knew that I was delivering a devastating blow to her and then offering some small ray of hope with treatment. I wrote her a prescription for the shots she would learn to self-administer. However, she called later that day to tell me that she could not pay the $800-per-month copay that the insurance company had imposed on this MS drug. There were no cheaper or generic drugs and no alternative treatments available, so she simply had to go without, even though she had "good" health insurance. Despite letters and phone calls from me to the insurance company, I was unable to help her. Over the next year she suffered several more MS exacerbations that landed her in the hospital, which cost the insurance company more than the preventative treatment would have and left my patient in worsening condition, and eventually on disability. She did not qualify for help from the pharmaceutical company because she had insurance. It is not surprising that the insurance company dropped her coverage, and after a long battle she got social security and qualified for Medicare. Finally, she was able through public assistance to get her MS treatment, but by this time she was wheelchair-bound in a chronic, progressive state of MS, and the medication was no longer indicated. What good are treatments that patients cannot get? Physicians are often caught in the middle, battling for life-saving treatments for our patients, which is an infuriating, frustrating experience.

## INSURANCE COMPANIES' COSTS AND CONTROL OVER HEALTH CARE

The insurance companies are another major source of skyrocketing health-care costs. Every year, premiums are raised; physicians' payments are reduced, and are these companies profitable? You bet they are. Even with the stock market losses of the past few years, the insurance companies have stayed on top. Their lobbyists in government convince legislators to maintain the status quo, and their control and influence on medical care is alarming. They pass judgment daily on who will or will not receive treatments, tests, or medications that their doctors prescribe. They have the power of life or death over our patients and the power to drive physicians out of business by taking away their patients. The costs to physicians include malpractice or liability insurance, office liability insurance, and health insurance for themselves and their staff, all of which have risen year after year. On the other side of the equation, health insurance and Medicare/Medicaid reimbursement for services rendered is decreasing each year. With nearly fifty million people uninsured in America, more and more physicians and hospitals are providing care which will never be reimbursed. These factors cause physicians to work longer hours, seeing more patients for less pay, and at some point the last straw is reached, and physicians are driven out of practice.

Back in San Diego, a colleague of mine had gotten sick and tired of dealing with a large insurance company, so he canceled his network provider status. He was under the assumption that his longtime patients would remain loyal to him and pay a little extra to continue seeing him. Within a few months, however, he shut down his ophthalmology practice and moved out of state. He had no bargaining power as an individual, and collective bargaining is outlawed for individual physicians. The insurance company simply diverted the patients to another provider who was willing to accept their terms. His patients were not loyal to him, despite the excellent care he had provided over many years. All his patients on that insurance plan were simply diverted to another ophthalmology group that was willing to accept their terms.

Physicians deserve to be paid for their services in a timely way, don't they?

Physicians are spending too much unpaid time chasing down reimbursement for work they have done. Many companies are deliberately and intentionally withholding payments until the physicians and their office staff have exhausted all means of appeal. A recent AMA (American Medical Association) study showed that approximately 20 percent of all insurance claims submitted by physicians were denied for processing errors that delayed the physicians' payments or caused them to be rejected (Crane, 2011). Processing errors like these are costing physicians their practices, as they find themselves unable to meet their overhead expenses and are forced to close their doors. Many valid claims are never paid because the physician's staff gave up appealing their claims because it takes too much time. The insurance companies count on this. There's no telling how much money insurance companies are saving by not paying doctors for the care their clients (patients) have received.

The insurance companies do not reimburse physicians for the time they spend filling out mountains of forms to file a claim and the subsequent appeals. They pay only for the time spent directly with the patient. As patient advocates, we often find ourselves going to battle with the insurance companies to get tests approved or to get life-saving, state–of-the-art medications and treatments covered. All this extra effort on the patient's behalf is incredibly time-consuming for physicians and their office staff.

The insurance industry controls physicians both coming and going. Once we agree to health insurance provider status, we must agree to all the terms they dictate about payment and approval of tests and treatments we provide. We must rely on insurance companies for our livelihood and play by their rules for payment on claims. Most physicians have very little bargaining power when it comes to revision of the provider contracts we are expected to sign. Some large and prominent groups that perform services that are not readily available in a community do have some bargaining power, but primary care physicians, for example, whose services can more easily be replaced, are basically screwed.

A large neurosurgery group in our area had very little competition, and as a result they were able to negotiate better rates of pay, no preauthorization of tests they ordered, and prompt payment of claims.

In order to offer neurosurgery treatment to their "clients," the insurance company agreed not to interfere with the practices of these neurosurgeons. They got "Gold Card" status because they were bargaining as a group, and their services could not be replaced by other physicians in their community. Large, multispecialty groups that care for sizable segments of the community also have special bargaining power with the insurance companies. These reimbursement issues are some of the factors that are forcing solo private practice doctors out of business and into large group practices and hospital employment.

On the other end of the cost equation, we pay insurance companies for malpractice liability insurance to maintain our hospital privileges and insurance provider status. The insurance companies exert control over how, where, and when we practice. A neurosurgeon in Florida was restricted from covering the local hospital's emergency room or his malpractice coverage would be canceled. How would you feel if you were in a car accident and had a subdural hematoma that was life-threatening, and no neurosurgeon would come in to see you because his malpractice insurance carrier wouldn't let him? It happened to a young man—a husband and a father—in Jacksonville, Florida. When this trauma patient, who was involved in a motor vehicle accident in Jacksonville, Florida, was brought to the ER with an acute brain injury, he had to be transferred 200 miles away to be seen by a neurosurgeon! The neurosurgeon who used to cover the ER had to give up his privileges due to the malpractice insurance costs. By the time this patient was treated, he did not fare well. Had he been treated as soon as he arrived in the original hospital's ER, he would have had less permanent brain damage and perhaps even recovered completely normally.

Ob-Gyn physicians are being forced to give up delivering babies due to exorbitant or nonexistent malpractice insurance. A pregnant patient in Florida may have to travel over 200 miles to be seen by a obstetrician, but, as we all know, when it comes time to deliver a baby, a three- or four-hour ride in the car to the doctor is not only inconvenient, it is also unsafe, which forces more deliveries by non-specialists in emergency rooms and hallways, by physicians or nurse practitioners who know nothing of the patient or her prenatal care evaluations or issues.

These are simply a few examples of how the practice of medicine is going bad because of malpractice insurance companies making decisions on where and how physicians can or cannot practice their specialty because of malpractice concerns. These are not medical decisions based on the patient's best interests, but economic-risk-based decisions that insurance companies make all day long, which impede physicians from doing what they are trained to do, to take care of all patients that need them.

Insurance companies collectively control both the income and expense sides of the financial equation, and they are giving physicians the squeeze of their lives. If health insurance companies don't agree with how we practice, they can cut us off as providers and cut off the income we rely on from treating our patients. If we have malpractice lawsuits, they can cancel our malpractice insurance whether or not we were found guilty. If we practice in remote areas where physicians are so badly needed, we usually cannot see enough patients—or at least enough insured patients—to meet our overhead expenses. If we don't work diligently and put in long hours filled with patient encounters, we can't afford the insurance we are struggling to pay. Insurance companies have nearly total control over the rates they pay for their medical providers, whose only bargaining chip is to withdraw from provider contracts. We lose our patients when they switch to another provider who accepts their insurance payment rates. There are also no limits on the rates that insurance companies charge physicians for their malpractice insurance. The rates vary widely across the country, and, in some states, these rates have caused an exodus of physicians to more affordable malpractice regions (Hellinger et al., 2002). Florida, Pennsylvania, North Carolina, and New Jersey are states that physicians have left at an alarming rate. New physicians must consider malpractice insurance rates when deciding where to start up their practices.

There were many days when I felt like a mouse running on a wheel in a vicious cycle where only the insurance companies benefited. We physicians are paying most of the money we earn from one insurance company to another for malpractice liability, office liability, and health insurance. Unless things change, it will simply be a losing proposition to practice medicine at all. Who would want to work this hard and sacrifice so much, just to *pay* for the privilege of practicing medicine? There are many dedicated physicians out there, but the situation is deteriorating so rapidly, we cannot expect that they will remain in practice no matter how bad it gets.

# MANAGED CARE OR MIDDLEMAN

The third piece of the puzzle of rising health care costs involves managed care insurance companies. The original HMOs (health management or maintenance organizations) were nonprofit organizations set up for certain labor groups, like the mine workers. In the sixties, the first for-profit HMOs emerged, and they blossomed in the eighties. With promises of cheaper health insurance rates, they entice businesses and individuals to sign up. These for-profit companies collect advance payments from their enrollees, and dole out health care in a "managed way." They review and control practically every decision the physician makes that would cost them money, such as blood tests, radiology tests, and procedures like biopsy or surgery. They have certain criteria whereby they approve a test and deny the rest. However, they don't cover all situations that a physician encounters in real life and in real patients individually. Guidelines are just that. They are not strict rules or parameters that should replace assessment of the individual patient's clinical condition by their physician after a detailed history and physical examination. Tests and treatments are often denied inappropriately, leaving to the physician the responsibility of fighting for the patient to get authorization. The physician's office has to fill out forms, call and wait on hold for interminable amounts of time, and often fax they physician's office notes to the insurance company to get the authorization. Many of us suspect that the excessive paperwork and hoops we are made to jump through are designed simply to make us give up and forget about getting authorization for a test or treatment after the initial denial.

However, it is the physician or his or her staff who has to tell the patient and their family that the test they were just convinced was necessary was not approved. Appeals on their behalf, including having their doctor get on the phone and call the managed care company, were to no avail. We get to tell the patient that they could go without the test or pay for it themselves, if they have an extra $3,000 or so to spare, for an MRI or a CT scan. Doing without the added information might or might not make a difference, but it is still a position that physicians hate being placed in, and it adds to the stress of practicing under managed care rules.

Even worse, imagine having to tell your patient that they cannot get the life-changing or life-saving treatment that you know would help them because their insurance won't cover it. The patient and their family have no one else toward whom to direct their anger but the physician in front of them. Welcome to the world where physicians are repeatedly scorned and made to feel less competent, less efficient, and in need of micromanagement.

The bottom line is that the less the managed care insurance companies spend on their "clients," the bigger their profits. They are in business to make profits. They contract with physicians, who are called "providers," who are willing to accept their highly discounted fees. They call their patients "clients" or "customers." Like most insurance companies, they make their profits from people who are healthy and don't use their insurance for long periods or only have minor or preventative treatments. They have carte blanche rights to refuse coverage to people with chronic illnesses or deny coverage for specific preexisting conditions. They can even cancel an existing client's coverage after they get sick, which of course leaves them uninsurable by any company. They do this by finding some loophole in the original insurance application, such as a minor medical condition you forgot to report, to cancel the policy. If you find yourself without a job, there is a guarantee of the option to continue coverage called Cobra, but it is at rates that most people cannot afford, and after eighteen months, the rates go up to astronomical levels. When I became disabled, I was terminated from my position as assistant professor at a local university medical center. The Cobra health insurance rate was over $1,000 per month. Because my husband had recently suffered a heart attack, and I had a back injury that was now chronic, we were now uninsurable by any company. We had no choice but to scrape together this money from a dwindling savings, to continue the only insurance available to us. At the end of the eighteen-month period, the rates were to go up to $2,400 per month for my husband and $1,100 per month for me to continue the same coverage. Although I had been both a faithful patron of, and provider for, this large insurance company for years, there was no loyalty, no exception, no help of any kind. It was only because of good luck that we were able to find new jobs that accommodated our disabilities, and we were able to obtain group health insurance through my new employer, a radiology managed care organization, at more affordable rates. Being a physician did not shield me from life's situations or give me any special consideration from the corporate, business-minded mentality of the insurance companies whose goal is to insure healthy people and cancel the policies of the sick. A few years later, I lost my job after two more back surgeries. After the Cobra ran out, the rates for continuing coverage were up to $4,000 per month, and we were otherwise uninsurable. In an ironic twist of fate, we have now joined the ranks of the uninsured millions. We must remain uninsured for six months to qualify for our state's high risk insurance pool which will still cost nearly $1,000 per month. After devoting my life to the field of medicine, I am shut out from access to it. On the bright side, by 2014, my husband and I will be eligible, when preexisting conditions are no longer allowed by the Affordable Care Act as a reason to deny health care coverage. Yeah.

If people are members of an HMO, their physicians must be providers or, in many cases, they will not be paid at all. Specialists must obtain referrals from the patient's primary care physician (PCP) to see these patients. The PCPs are often penalized or "called on the carpet" for ordering too many referrals to specialists. Once the patient is seen, his or her insurance must be factored in before ordering any tests. These tests frequently require preauthorization, which can take days or weeks and require reams of paperwork. There are different management groups physicians may have to contact for radiology testing, pharmaceutical benefits, or procedures like surgery for one patient's care. For one individual patient, three or more calls and forms may be required before anything can be done for the patient! The insurance may not completely cover the tests or treatments, in which case the patient may have to pay a percentage of the cost. It is usually the physician's office staff who has to explain the cost breakdown to the patient, with no remuneration for the time and effort they went through to get an authorization. When writing prescriptions, physicians must be sure that the medication they wish to prescribe is on the specific formulary for a particular insurance company. There are hundreds of different insurance plans and companies with different permutations of the coverage rules. It may seem like a good idea for consumers and employers to be able to pick a plan according to the rates and variable coverage, although no one can predict whether they will need coverage for a bone marrow transplant or specialized treatment for a brain tumor. When they find that the plan with a cheaper premium doesn't cover the high-cost but medically necessary treatment they need, it can lead to major problems both for the patient and for the physician, who no longer has all the tools necessary to maximize his or her patient's chances of survival.

Dealing with insurance companies and these various managed-care organizations makes the physician's job almost impossible. It's like keeping track of all the choices on a Chinese menu. You have one option from column A and two from column B. To keep all these insurance factors in mind while trying to deliver the best-quality medical care to each patient is not something they taught us in medical school or residency, and the frustration levels of physicians are rising exponentially because of it. We rely on our office staff to understand and handle much of the paperwork, but if a mistake is made, the responsibility falls back on us.

An example of the ridiculous nature of our so-called competitive society is that governmental regulations forbid insurance companies from selling health insurance products across state lines, thus ensuring them free rein to uncontrolled, monopolistic rate increases. Is this an example of how the capitalistic model works to the benefit of the people, promoting competition and free markets?

The incentives are all wrong in the managed care system, because the less that the administrators of these plans spend on actual patient care, the more they get to keep in profits. They reward the doctors who spend the least on patient care while seeing the most patients. They punish the primary care doctors who spend more on their patients for treatments, tests or referrals to specialists. They punish doctors who spend more time with their patients, by devaluing the reimbursement. I have had several colleagues who were dumped by HMOs for ordering too many tests or specialty referrals. Many people can recall times when their primary care doctor refused to refer them to a specialist or to order a test for their symptoms. The term "gatekeepers" has been applied to primary care doctors by the managed care organizations, and this was meant to be a compliment! While the primary physician may truly feel the problem is not complex or severe enough to warrant the extra workup or referral, there are frequently economic reasons for this, not medical ones, dictated by the HMOs. Physicians are continually being asked to compromise their standards of patient care for the benefit of managed care organizations. It can certainly be an uphill battle not to cave in to the demands of the managed care companies.

As I mentioned earlier, when I went into private practice in San Diego, I naively signed up with nearly all the managed care plans in the area. I knew little or nothing about these companies, and reading through their contracts was like taking a massive dose of sedatives. I had never learned "Legalese." I only knew that without their patients I would not have sufficient numbers of patients to keep my practice busy. I admit that I indiscriminately signed up with every company that offered me the opportunity, although these contracts were essentially nonnegotiable anyway. This helped me get plenty of patients, but I soon realized that many of these companies were not honoring their part of the bargain. They were withholding care by denying proposed tests or treatments. They were withholding payment for the work their physician providers had done. Several of the Tenncare (Tennessee's Medicaid) managed care groups have run similar scams. They go bankrupt or dissolve their businesses, leaving the providers unpaid. Yet somehow the administrators of these plans see very big profits and salaries. At one point in my career, I signed up with the Blue Cross network. I saw hundreds of BlueCare (Tennessee Medicaid managed by Blue Cross) patients over an eight-month period, with all the appropriate referrals. Blue Cross denied payment because they told me I was never assigned a provider number. Although they had my universal Blue Cross provider application, and approved each individual patient's visits, a failure on their part to assign me a number was their justification to refuse payment for the hundreds of hours of work I did caring for their enrollees. I lost about $80,000 in that rip-off. Is it any wonder I stopped seeing TennCare patients after that? There is a limit to anyone's willingness to help out with disabled and disadvantaged patients. This is especially true now that physicians are having a tough time paying their basic overhead. After being refused payment for the hard work we've done over and over again, it is understandable that many physicians just want out of the rat race.

People want access to the best-quality health care available today. They want to be free to choose their own physicians. A backlash against managed care in the nineties closed down most of the HMOs. In their place, PPOs (preferred provider organizations) rose up to prominence. They were less restrictive, although patients would still have to pay extra to see a doctor who wasn't on the provider list. They were still subject to denials for medications or treatments their doctors recommended, if someone in the company deemed the treatment unnecessary or "investigational."

After the medical profession had used IVIG, a purified blood product for myasthenia gravis, for fifteen years, with hundreds of publications—even textbooks—recommending it as an effective therapy for those patients who find themselves in serious trouble with this disease, Blue Cross of Tennessee refused to cover it by calling it "investigational." Amazingly, this medication was an accepted standard of care and covered by Blue Cross of Kentucky and most other states, as well as by other insurance companies, for exacerbations of myasthenia gravis. I had a patient with myasthenia gravis who was also a diabetic, and he needed this treatment to keep his disease under control. The only other choice I had was to hospitalize him for plasmapheresis, a much more invasive and risky treatment, or to treat him with IVIG in the hospital and hope that he would not get stuck with the bill. The other treatments, such as steroids and other immune-suppressing medications, are fraught with side effects, especially for diabetics. They not only put the patient at risk for infections, they can also cause the patient's blood sugar to rise out of control. My patient's insurance company refused to pay for IVIG because it's so expensive. I wrote a letter of appeal to the company, which should have carried some weight, in light of my position as an assistant professor in a top university medical school, and a subspecialist in treating this disease. It was again denied. I was instructed to speak to a physician representative, on the phone, which I did next. After my narrative summary of the patient's case, and after I cited several references regarding this life-saving treatment's effectiveness, the physician with whom I was speaking said, "I am a family practice physician. I don't know anything about that disease. Anyway, I can't approve this—you'll have to fill out a form and send it to the board in Chattanooga."

So, I got the form, filled it out, attached over twenty references and a book citation, and guess what? Turned down again. The rejection letter I got gave me the alternative of an arbitration hearing. Not only would I have had to continue donating my time for this patient's cause, I would have had to pay a minimum of $150.00 for the arbitration fee and more money for each hour that the hearings went on. At that point I finally gave up, which was exactly what these companies count on. They figured out that if you make the appeal process cumbersome enough for physicians and leave no option for the individual patient without the help of their physician to appeal these kinds of economically driven decisions, they will eventually do something else to treat the patient. In this case, I admitted the patient to the hospital, where I did not have to get prior authorization for individual medications, and treated the patient with the IVIG he needed, which cost the insurance company not only the cost of the medication but also a five-day hospital stay. In the end the patient got better, and we averted the impending crisis that could have led to his requiring a ventilator, or breathing machine, to survive, and he was able to go home and resume his normal life. The satisfaction that I had done a good deed for this patient was the only reimbursement I got for all the extra hours of frustration I put into dealing with his insurance company while providing for his care and treatment. It would seem that this is what being a physician is all about these days.

Our local and national medical societies seem to be relatively impotent to battle the kinds of injustices that go on in the insurance industry on a daily basis. I wonder if there are many other professions that go to bat for their "clients" the way we do, without remuneration of any kind. The pharmaceutical companies love it; we line their pockets with our efforts to get an expensive, nonformulary, brand-name medication approved for our patient's use. If we were lawyers, we would get rich charging for the time spent on each patient outside of the office visit. Our medical records, prepared each day for each patient, are the legal documents that lawyers use for their cases. These records are examined by the insurance companies and Medicare for fraud or abuse in our reimbursement systems. Throughout our careers we are reminded that if it wasn't documented, it wasn't done. Being a good writer is as important these days as being a compassionate, competent physician.

Physicians are losing the battle against corporate medicine and closing their doors to seek alternative careers or to delegate the responsibility of dealing with insurance companies to others. We are witnessing the death of the private-practice physician, and perhaps the death of the doctor-patient relationship, and I, for one, am saddened by this. The value lost may be intangible to many who see physicians as a commodity in the health-care picture or as unruly children needing strict supervision, but from the other end of the stethoscope, the medical profession is being suffocated by micromanagement and excessive paperwork.

The physicians who are contracted providers have accepted lower and lower reimbursement rates, yet insurance premiums have seen double-digit increases in the past three years. Profit margins for managed care companies have increased from1.9 percent in 1999 to

4.4 percent in 2002 and 6.2 percent in 2007 (CNN Money, 2008). This amounts to billions of dollars, which is paid for by the people, and the rewards are reaped by a small group of administrators. By denying expensive treatments or medications to enrollees and cutting down on payments to their providers, they save more money for their own profits. They entice employers by promising lower rates but deliver lower reimbursement to physicians and hospitals, with frequent denials for payment. Double-digit increases in premium rates, however, have made many employers drop insurance coverage entirely. The percentage of people covered by employment-based health insurance decreased in 2010 to 55 percent. The percentage of people covered by any type of private health insurance has been dropping since 2001, while the number of people on Medicaid or Medicare has increased, according to the U.S. Census Bureau (U.S. Census Bureau, 2010). Employers that do provide health-insurance benefits have been passing more of the costs on to their employees over the last nine years. In a study by the Milliman Medical Index, the total cost of healthcare for a family of four in 2011 averaged $19,393, compared to $9,235 in 2002 (Mayne et al., 2011). Because of this, we have a huge number of working people in this country who have no insurance coverage. Even physicians are often unable to provide insurance benefits to their employees, as the cost has skyrocketed.

The number of Americans without health insurance has risen steadily over the years and is now over fifty million (U.S. Census Bureau, 2010). These uninsured people are not immune to having medical problems; in fact they are often some of the sickest patients we see. An estimated 45,000 people die each year for lack of health insurance (Wilper, et al., 2009). Although they may be sick, they avoid going to the hospital because they know they can't afford to, and don't want to burden their families. An estimated 11.4 million people with chronic illness like diabetes, hypertension and high cholesterol cannot get insurance (Wilper, et al., 2008). When people end up in the ER with a catastrophic illness, they know they cannot pay the tens of thousands of dollars their hospital bills will be. Medical bills were the primary reason for bankruptcy filings in this country in 2009. What is even more shocking is that most of the people surveyed in this study had health insurance, but the copays, deductibles, and noncovered expenses in their plans led them to bankruptcy anyway, if their illness was long or severe enough. Severe illness led them to lose their jobs and insurance coverage, so they eventually ended up uninsured and bankrupt as well (Tamkins, 2009).The uninsured in general are not a wealthy group and usually do not end up paying for their medical care. Who pays for the health care of the uninsured? Doctors and hospitals and, in some cases, charity organizations do.

Physicians have learned a hard lesson since the advent of HMOs. There is no loyalty among our patients when it comes to paying for their medical care. Physicians, who once had patients whom they followed for years and even over generations within a family, now realize that in our current system, they are as expendable as a used car. People switch doctors and expect the same quality of care from a physician who just met them for the first time as they did from a physician who knew them for years. The switch is more often than not to the result of a change in insurance. The relationship between doctor and patient may not be considered important or of any added value by the insurance or managed care companies, but in reality, it makes a big difference in the quality and cost of medical care. For example, a young woman was under a great deal of stress at home and in her job. She would experience this stress in physical ways with symptoms like chest pressure, shortness of breath, numbness and tingling of her fingers, and a sense of impending doom. Her longtime physician knew from prior screening exams and his relationship with her that these symptoms were anxiety related and treated her with gentle reassurance and medications for anxiety. Her job switched insurance plans to an HMO, and her physician was not a contracted provider. She got a new physician, who saw her in a ten-minute visit, heard the complaints she voiced, and because he didn't have time even to inquire about her personal situation, he simply acted on the symptoms she described. He referred her to a cardiologist, a pulmonary specialist, and a neurologist. She underwent a cardiac stress test, an EKG and an echocardiogram, pulmonary function tests, chest X-rays, nerve conduction tests, blood tests, and MRI scans of her brain and spine. In the end, all these tests were normal, but by now the patient's anxiety level had risen to an extreme level. Since all these doctors seemed to be convinced that she was seriously ill and ordered all of these tests on her heart, lungs, and brain, she also began to believe that there was really something major wrong with her. This exacerbated her anxiety symptoms and led her to search the Internet and seek more medical opinions to determine the cause. The cost of these additional physician charges, tests, and unnecessary medicines rose into the thousands of dollars and only worsened her underlying anxiety. Is it possible that her original physician would have missed some serious problem, which manifested itself in those symptoms? Yes, but the patient had responded to reassurance and treatment for her anxiety previously, making the additional workup unnecessary, and if her symptoms persisted, she could have communicated that with her longtime physician, and he could then have arranged for additional tests, or perhaps a psychiatric evaluation. In a close, long-term doctor-patient relationship, physicians remember their patients and the kinds of problems they have had, previous medication reactions or treatment failures, and previous tests that have been done to rule in or out serious illnesses. They are more likely to recognize a new problem that may require further workup. They get to know their patient's personality and how he or she reacts to illness or pain. They have records of previous visits and test results. Every time patients switch physicians, they start over with a blank slate—a stranger—and this ends up costing patients and insurance companies more. More important, the trust, intimacy and communication between patient and physician that has been built up over time is lost.

Managed care is the main reason for early retirement cited by physicians over fifty (Greene, 2000). These older physicians are retiring at an alarming rate, more so than at any other time in history. According to a survey in the year 2000 by Merritt, Hawkins and Associates, a national physician search and consulting firm, 38 percent of physicians planned to retire within the next one to three years. Another 10 percent planned to seek employment in a nonclinical setting (Merritt, Hawkins and Associates, 2000). Not only is managed care reducing the quality of patient care in this country, the frustration of doctors who try to deal with these companies is causing them to get out of medicine altogether. The loss of physicians in practice is reducing the availability of medical care as well. Health care centers on physicians. Without them, there is no one left to administer health care. When we lose a physician because he or she can no longer put up with the frustration of dealing with managed care or malpractice issues, our society loses a chance of providing universal health care to our population, and it is a tragedy for all. We hasten the day when a severe shortage of physicians will occur, as has been predicted by the Council on Graduate Medical Education (Iglehart, 2010).

At the same time, medical care is more flawed now than ever before and needs some form of quality control. There must be some form of oversight and some way of controlling health care costs. There are several reasons for this. First of all, physicians are imperfect and subject to errors of omission and commission just like any human being. Most physicians can remember a colleague whose competence they wondered about, who may have missed an obvious diagnosis, or who injured a patient through their lack of action. When you are asked to get involved in a botched case, it can be a very difficult situation to maneuver through without doing more damage.

There has been an unwritten code—like a fraternal order—that most physicians have learned to live by, to protect each other and our careers before our patients. This is because the risk of reporting an error or bad outcome is so great. Reports of errors end up in lawyers' hands, and physicians risk losing their livelihoods if the error is discovered by a malpractice trial lawyer. The hospital they practice in may curtail or revoke their attending privileges. An insurance company may cancel their provider status. In a survey by the Agency for Healthcare Research and Quality, over 1,000 physicians surveyed were willing to report error information if it would be kept confidential and non-discoverable by lawyers, and if the information would be used to improve the system and not for punitive action (Agency for HealthCare Research and Quality, 2008).

Many physicians have developed flawed practice styles that are based on personal experience rather than evidence-based medicine. Sometimes I would see three patients with a rare diagnosis clustered in one day or week, and soon I started looking for that diagnosis in everybody. Even though it was statistically unlikely, and I might not see another patient with that diagnosis again for a year or two, the personal experience of recent times clouded my judgment for a time. Does it make sense for me to keep ordering an expensive test for a rare disease on every patient just because of my experience with three individuals? Similarly, a physician who gets burned in a lawsuit for missing some rare disease in one patient will forever change his or her practice habits, ordering more tests that are probably unnecessary in order to avoid missing a rare diagnosis again.

Unfortunately, there are also less honorable reasons for some of the million-dollar workups some patients get. There are often secondary gain issues for physicians who own expensive radiology testing equipment or labs and who order more tests than necessary in order to pay for their investment. Through the process of self-referral, an entrepreneurial physician can become an unethical physician in the blink of an eye. Greed is unfortunately a factor in many physicians' medical decision-making process. A small group of physicians simply are lazy about maintaining the diligence necessary to their practices. It is quicker and easier to order a CT scan on every patient who has a bellyache than to do a detailed history and examination, form a differential diagnosis, and treat the most likely diagnosis conservatively, before considering expensive tests that also expose the patient to radiation. It is easier to give a prescription for pain pills than to argue with a patient about the need for narcotics or to urge the person to try alternative approaches.

Of course, as in many occupations, there are just a handful of physicians who are ruining the practice of medicine for the rest and forcing more regulation and restrictions on free practice choices for physicians. There is a need for more uniform practice guidelines and standards of care that are overseen and enforced by a panel of our peers. Rather than expert witnesses, we should have more expert panels, and less risk associated with reporting or correcting a problem for an individual physician who finds themselves or a colleague in the wrong. We need to adopt more backup systems to help avoid errors such as the mistakes that can lead to operations on the wrong limb or mistaken doses of medications. We spend so much time and money attacking physicians who have made mistakes rather than spending our resources identifying and correcting problems as they come up in a more preventative approach, while not sacrificing the entire careers of physicians who stray from practice standards. If we take away the incentives for physicians to veer away from quality health care before profits or fear, we can steer ourselves away from the brink of chaos in medicine.

Unfortunately, the people who are currently doing the oversight and quality control are the ones who hold the pocketbook—the insurance companies. Their bottom line is the standard by which many of the medical decisions are measured. Having worked in the medical management field, I can tell you that most of the physicians who sit on these panels are a very dedicated, informed, and concerned group. However, they often have very limited and incomplete documentation from the treating physicians to work with when making the decisions about medical treatments or imaging studies for a given patient. There are often circumstances that are unknown to the managed care reviewers that would make a difference in approval of a test or treatment. There are systems in place to appeal these decisions, but they take up more time and cause more difficulties for the practicing physician. In addition, the physicians on these managed care panels have limited authority to make policy decisions within these companies. The administrative departments pull all the strings and take home the big bucks, and their decisions are based on one thing: profits.

## LAWYERS AND HEALTH CARE COSTS

Lawyers play a large role in causing the escalation of health care costs. Malpractice claims have not only been increasing in number, but the amounts of jury awards have become extravagant, as well. The lawyers keep anywhere from 30 to 40 percent of a successful verdict award, and this can amount to millions for a single successful case they litigate. Incentives like these have a tendency to raise the rates of cases without merit, the so-called frivolous lawsuits being filed. It is easy to understand the motivation to sue a doctor, in the hopes of a successful verdict that will provide the patients and their lawyers with instant riches. This has had a twofold effect on costs. The malpractice liability insurance companies raise their rates for doctors, and doctors learn to practice "defensive medicine."

Physicians' malpractice liability insurance rates have gotten out of control, doubling and even tripling in just the past several years. In some states, the rates are simply unaffordable under any circumstances and physicians are moving to other states that have lower rates. Insurance companies report spending tens of billions of dollars in defending and paying out legal expenses. Thirty billion dollars could go a long way toward providing everyone in this country with top-quality health care. The malpractice issues that are crippling America's physicians are discussed more thoroughly in Chapter 4.

## RISING OVERHEAD COSTS

In most businesses, there is a bottom line. In order to survive, one must consider profits, losses, and cost containment, and adjust one's business plan accordingly. In a normal business, when costs go up, prices go up in order to keep a business profitable. In the business of medicine, there is very little control over costs or reimbursement for services rendered. The only choice a physician has is to increase their workload in order to be profitable. This means that physicians are seeing more patients in less time and working longer hours every day. Physicians have to cut corners in the quality of care they deliver to their patients when a visit goes from twenty minutes to five. It is difficult to get to the root of a problem in five minutes, so physicians rely on more tests, instead of taking a careful history and doing a thorough physical exam. It is easier for physicians to order more tests than to rely on their diagnostic skills or those of their assistants. Patients nowadays expect to have the expensive tests anyway. They go online, and they watch medical TV shows. They have just enough medical knowledge to be dangerous. Many people have lost confidence in their physicians' abilities to diagnose and treat their conditions properly. With the constant threat of malpractice lawsuits, physicians dare not take a chance on missing anything, however unlikely or rare it may be. However, all these unnecessary tests are raising the costs we all pay for health care today. Since physicians are also patients and must pay for their own health insurance and that of their families and staff, if possible, they are contributing to the rising cost of their own overhead.

So, just what do physicians pay for their overhead? The costs of running a private medical practice vary tremendously according to the specialty and location. I can give some estimates based on my experience as a neurologist. The overhead that a physician shells out each month begins with the office rental or mortgage payment. This is usually quite a bit more expensive than a house payment. A rough estimate is $2,000–$3,000 a month per physician in an average office near a medical center or hospital. The office decor may be simple or extravagant, and these costs can run up the overhead as well. The employees' salaries may run $8,000–$10,000 dollars a month, for an office manager, a nurse, and a receptionist—the basics for a physician. If there is a billing service, they typically charge 6 to 8 percent of collections, which could run from $1,500 to $1,800 per month. Then there are the costs of equipment. Office equipment like the computers and medical practice software that allows for scheduling, billing, and storing the financial information for the practice may run another $1,000 per month. Recently, legislation has made it a requirement to have an Electronic Medical Record system to store and transmit records among colleagues, hospitals, and insurance companies. The cost of these programs is high—in the tens of thousands of dollars—although the federal government has some tax credits available for their implementation. Copiers, fax machines, stationary, medical transcription, charts, and other office supplies make up another large portion of the overhead, which average another $1,000 per month. Communications, including the costs of telephone systems with several lines, answering systems and intercoms, pagers and cell phones, average another $1,000 per month. Besides office equipment, most physicians have medical equipment that may be needed to practice their specialty. From EKGs to ultrasound, this equipment is expensive, and payments on equipment may add a minimum of a $1,000 per month to the overhead. Insurance costs, of course, make up a huge part of the overhead. Malpractice insurance costs have doubled, tripled, or even quadrupled in the last several years. The amounts range from $6,000 per year in rural areas with low malpractice incidents in low risk specialties to more than $200,000 per year for high-risk specialties like obstetrics and neurosurgery in states like Florida, where the incidence of malpractice lawsuits is high. In addition, there is liability insurance for the office, umbrella liability coverage for the physician, worker's compensation for the employees, health insurance for the physician and his or her employees, insurance on the office and equipment, auto insurance, life insurance, disability insurance, and on and on. An average monthly total for this neurologist would be approximately $5,000.

Like many other small businesses in this country, health insurance costs are threatening to bankrupt physicians. We are forced to make tough choices, like whether even to offer health insurance to our employees. I'm ashamed to say that many physicians' offices do not. There are also taxes, which include business taxes, employment taxes and income tax, social security tax, and Medicare tax. Approximately 40 percent of our gross income is paid out in taxes. The amount of tax depends on the income of the physician and the number of employees, but for an average neurologist, taxes run about $3,000 per month. There are legal and accounting costs that can vary tremendously, depending on whether the business is incorporated or whether there are specific legal issues being dealt with. On average, however, a low estimate of these costs would be $500 per month. In order to maintain one's professional license and certification, specialty society dues and continuing medical education are required. Physicians must attend annual meetings and take additional training courses every year in order to keep current on the latest medical information or techniques that apply to their specialty. These costs include traveling to and from annual society meetings, membership dues, books, journals, and more recently, online continuing medical education courses. An average estimate for these costs would be in the range of $500 per month when two or three seminars per year are divided up. Overall, it is not uncommon for the direct overhead of a single physician these days to exceed $20,000 per month. If we divide this amount into the time the office is open and running, an average of forty hours per week, the cost of maintaining an office practice has risen to approximately $125 per hour! How many patients does a doctor have to see every hour to cover these costs? How many more to make a decent salary? These overhead costs must be paid first, and then the physician gets what's left over. The final slice of the physician's pie is down to about 10 percent of their overall collections, and it continues to decline.

Many physicians are trying to contain these costs by cutting back on insurance coverage, salaries, expensive equipment, and whatever else they can, but despite their best efforts, the overhead keeps going up. This is why so few physicians are opting for private practice these days. The additional hours spent running the business aspects of a practice can be a full-time job, in addition to patient care. The cost and complexity of compliance with the new regulations is becoming so burdensome that most private-practice physicians don't have the capital, time, or technical resources to do it. By the time the overhead and income taxes are paid, there is often little time or money left over, and for most physicians it just isn't worth it anymore. However, the loss of autonomy among hospital- or HMO-employed physicians is another source of great frustration and another reason for early retirement. I know I didn't spend half my life training to be a doctor just to end up as some corporation's employee, answering to an administrator for each penny earned or spent in my business or on my patients, and carrying on the unfair practices of these corporations.

For many physicians, the employment model does work better, as less time is spent attending to business or making the difficult decisions that affect the bottom line. Somehow, physicians often feel their identity should be separate from the money part of their practices; they try not to let money color their ethical and moral judgment when it comes to medicine, although they are just closing their eyes to the ugly facts of for-profit health care. Ours is a hallowed and sacred occupation, something which has been forgotten in recent years. It used to be rare that a physician would refuse to see a patient regardless of their insurance or lack thereof. I never used to even ask about insurance coverage when I was called to see a patient. After enough refusals by insurance companies to pay for services rendered, however, it became hard to pay the overhead. Now, when one calls a physician's clinic for an appointment, the first question is, "What's the patient's insurance?" If the patient has none, or if the doctor is not a "Provider," the ER at the county hospital, where no patient can be refused, becomes the primary care doctor's office, at great cost to all of us. As you can see, physicians are unable to control most of their overhead costs, which continue to rise annually, or their income, causing a greater dropout of physicians from medicine, and especially, from private practice.

## DECREASING REIMBURSEMENT RATES

The reimbursement rates for practicing medicine vary widely. It is meaningless to speak about what physicians charge for their care. Our so-called "usual and customary" charges are almost never what we actually get paid for our services. We get paid what each insurance company decides to pay us, and those amounts are declining every year. Most physicians collect about 50 to 60 percent of what they charge. If you ever look at an Explanation of Benefits (EOB) from your insurance company after a doctor's visit, you will see a big difference between what was charged and what was actually paid. The difference is usually what is written off by the physician. The electronic bill submitted to Medicare or private insurance is very complex. A single mistake in Medicare documentation or billing can be interpreted as fraud by Medicare auditors and can lead to fines of $15,000 per occurrence or more.

So, for all the talk about it, how much do physicians actually make? The average income of a physician is $150,000 and declining, although the range is very broad. When you calculate the eighty- to one-hundred-hour weeks they work, for eleven months per year, this comes out between $25 and $30 per hour. They are often the sole breadwinners of families, often supporting extended families as well.

Surgeons and other specialists who primarily do procedures tend to make much more than primary care doctors, and some physicians like pediatricians and family practitioners tend to make even less, despite how hard they work. The reimbursement for routine office visits is very poor, compared to surgery, procedures, or testing. Unfortunately, this and the time constraints that physicians are under to see more patients per day, have led to a greater reliance on testing and procedures, rather than the old-fashioned history and physical examinations. The devaluation of time spent with patients—taking histories, examining them, and discussing treatment—is a large part of the problem, especially for primary care, neurology, and psychiatry specialists. The incentives to do more procedures, tests, and surgeries and to see more patients in less time are where the big financial rewards exist in our current system. Even patients seem to have less confidence in their physicians and want tests to verify or disprove their physicians' diagnoses. The erosion of the doctor-patient relationship therefore contributes to the increase in cost of health care as well.

How physicians get paid involves a very complicated formula called RVUs or Relative Value Units, which the government created for the Medicare system. After all these years, I still can't make much sense of RVUs, but among the principles is that various geographical areas and different types of office visits have different "values." In other words, where a physician practices makes a difference in how much he or she is paid for Medicare patients.

Documentation of each visit and its "complexity" involves listing aspects of the history, including a review of systems, to qualify for higher reimbursement. The review of systems is when the doctor lists a number of conditions, such as heart disease or lung or kidney problems, and asks if you have had any of them. It is meant to uncover any conditions that may have been missed in the rest of the history and that may affect the diagnosis or treatment. Sometimes it is relevant, often it is not, and often it is the extra time necessary to discuss the primary complaint that matters to the physician and the patient, although not reimbursable by the Center for Medicare and Medicaid Services (CMS).

Different types of office visits, procedures, and other services all go into a pot, matched up with diagnosis codes called CPT codes. The Center for Medicare and Medicaid Services takes these complex formulas and decides how much to pay. There has been no accounting for the rising costs of overhead in these calculations by Medicare. In fact the plan has been to reduce the payment rates by a percentage, year after year. The Omnibus Budget Reconciliation Act of 1989 made changes to physician payments under Medicare. First it introduced the Medicare Fee Schedule, which took effect in 1992. Second, it limited the amount Medicare nonproviders could balance bill Medicare beneficiaries. Third, it introduced the Medicare Volume Performance Standards (MVPS) as a way to control costs. Physician reimbursement has been scheduled to go down 4–5 percent per year, based on these complex formulas. They call this the SGR, or sustainable growth rate, which is really an oxymoron when you think about it.

Each year physicians lobby and beg their congressmen to hold the rates steady for one more year. However, the deferred rate decrease has been added on to the next year's decrease, so that in 2012, the rate decrease is set to be nearly 30 percent. So, while the cost of running a practice has gone up, the reimbursement rates have indeed gone down. The commercial insurance companies have jumped on the bandwagon and reduced their reimbursement rates in line with the amounts that Medicare set. They typically pay a percentage—now 103 or 104 percent of the Medicare rate—which is much lower than most physicians actually charge for their services. Needless to say, reimbursement for all services has gone down or stayed flat over the past five years, as overhead has gone up, putting the pinch on physicians. There is no value in these reimbursement schemes for skill as a physician or for time taken to talk to patients and their families. Quality of care has not been recognized or rewarded. Higher numbers of patients and procedures are rewarded in the current fee-for-service system. Only time spent with the patient, which must be very well documented, is reimbursed. The time taken to review labs or X-rays or to call patients or their families is not reimbursed. Those of us whose specialties take up more time spent with each patient are punished in this procedure-oriented system. Those physicians who do not write extensive notes to document the visit with the patient are penalized and may be subject to audit and fines in this system. Medicare audits can be extremely costly for any discrepancy they find in documentation of a patient visit versus the codes the physician charged.

There are some promising changes underway, which include better reimbursement for primary care physicians, and quality guidelines that are meant to recognize those physicians who adhere to accepted standards of practice, where they have been defined. However, Neurology and Psychiatry are not included in these payment increases. Nevertheless, there is still a long way to go in rewarding and recognizing good physicians who take the time to foster a strong doctor-patient relationship, while doing their main diagnosis and healing treatments without expensive tests or procedures.

Physicians write off hundreds of thousands of dollars every year in uncollectible debts for uninsured patients, discounted reimbursements, and denials of claims by insurance companies and Medicare or Medicaid. Unlike other businesses, however, they are not allowed to declare any losses on their taxes for services provided that were never paid for. In the past few years, most insurance companies have reduced their payments toward the Medicare rates, and Medicare reimbursement rates have gone down by about 50 percent in the last ten years. Medicaid and its variations like the HMO-Medicaid programs pay about 25 per cent of physicians' customary charges. Reimbursement rates overall have gone down by about 25 percent in the past five years, as the overhead has gone up by at least that much.

Most physicians have little choice but to be providers for the major insurance companies, including Medicare, and accept their discounted rates. They have very little negotiating power as single physicians because if they choose not to be providers, their competition will, and they won't have enough patients coming through their doors. However, fewer and fewer physicians are accepting Medicaid or its state-based managed care counterparts like Tenncare or MediCal because of problems with reimbursement and difficulties in getting patients the type of care they need. Most physicians will tell you that they lose money on these Medicaid patients, since the overhead is higher than the reimbursement for the time spent. It is an ethical dilemma for a physician to refuse care to someone based on his or her insurance coverage. However, losing the business because we cannot pay the overhead would deny care to all our patients. We have been forced to make difficult choices that we don't like, but they are necessary for our survival as a profession. We cannot afford to take care of all the nations' fifty plus million uninsured or underinsured patients.

Powerful insurance company lobbyists have helped get laws put in place that prevent physicians from any collective bargaining. Can we refuse to accept an insurance company's rates of reimbursement? Sure we can, but only individually, not as a group. Collective bargaining as a group is strictly forbidden to physicians, who are not even allowed to compare their charges and reimbursements or agree on what usual and customary charges should be. However, powerful insurance companies who have control over thousands of patients can get together and fix prices as a group. They hold the doctors, the hospitals, and the patients in the palms of their hands. If we refuse to accept the terms of a given insurance company, then the patients on that plan will be switched to another physician who is a provider. Patients will accept the change in physicians to avoid having to pay extra for their care. The physicians who refuse to accept the insurance fee schedules will have no patients coming through their doors. This will simply hasten the day when we close our doors permanently. The divide-and-conquer philosophy has been applied to physicians, pitting them against each other so that these unfair insurance practices can be maintained. There is no transparency in these dealings with physicians and groups. Favoritism and special treatment are rampant, especially when it comes to physicians within certain specialties. The solo practitioner has the least bargaining power and is being forced out of business in favor of the large groups and hospital-employed practices.

If one physician refuses to accept reduced rates of payment, they simply lose the patients and their business. The patients are diverted to another physician willing to accept the terms dictated by insurance companies. Similarly, patients have no say in the rates they are expected to pay for health insurance. As the rates have gone up by double digits these past few years, we have been powerless to negotiate these rates with the insurance companies. The question about the patients enrolled in these large insurance company groups is only to have or have not. Recently, more and more physicians are refusing to see Medicare patients or limiting their Medicare patient numbers to stay afloat. The rates of reimbursement for an office visit or simple procedure are lower than the cost of overhead for many physicians, which makes even Medicare charity work. Medicaid has in fact been charity work for most physicians for years. The fee schedule for Medicare is skewed toward specialists who perform surgery, procedures or do radiologic interpretation. Legislation to improve reimbursement to primary care physicians is meant to encourage more graduates to choose these fields but does not include the cognitive work that physicians in neurology and psychiatry do each day, as we spend time actually talking to our patients and examining them thoroughly.

Overall, physicians who used to be more concerned with patient care have to worry about their bottom line, and whether they will be able to keep their doors open. Physicians in private practice are quickly becoming extinct, as they end up joining large, managed-care groups to survive. They give up not only their independence but also a great deal of the decision-making process in providing the best-quality care for their patients. They are now employees, supervised and reviewed each month by the administrators of these large groups. They are often forced to abide by regulations set up by people whose primary goal is making money, not the good of any individual patient. They are evaluated not on quality but on quantity and are often pressured to see more patients in less time, and to order the cheapest treatments, the fewest tests and referrals. The primary care physicians are discouraged from ordering expensive tests or referring patients to specialists. They are evaluated monthly and reprimanded or even fired if they spend too much money on their patients' care. Why? Because this takes money out of the CEO and administrator's pockets. The doctors who take a little extra time counseling their patients, who leave no stone unturned in making a difficult diagnosis, or who keep their patients in the hospital an extra day to make sure they can make it at home safely; these are the doctors who are penalized in this system.

Many physicians are uncomfortable with their role as businessmen or women. We were trained to practice medicine, and to consider our patients' welfare above all else, especially whether the patient can pay for their treatment. There are some physicians who have become very good at turning a profit and have mastered the business side of medicine. The emphasis is placed on quantity of patients seen, with many physicians pulling eighty- to one-hundred-hour work weeks, hiring "physician extenders" like nurse practitioners or physician assistants, or hiring other physicians at relatively low salaries and working them hard enough to turn a profit. Higher-paid tests and procedures are emphasized rather than traditional one-on-one patient evaluation and management, which are underpaid for the amount of time involved under the current insurance reimbursement system. However, it is hard to be good at both the business and the art of medicine. The quality of medical care and the doctor-patient relationship are inevitably sacrificed when patients are whisked through their doctor's visit or are not even seen by a doctor at all.

Unfortunately, there are also a lot of cutthroat competitive business dealings in the medical community. Physicians in large communities compete with one another. Physician employees in medical groups are often used, abused, and cheated out of their earnings. They are often recruited to jobs with empty promises of ideal practice conditions and great salaries. It is impossible to understand the real situation in a practice setting until you get there and start working. When you join a group of physicians, it is like getting married to people to whom you were just introduced. You are going to be spending a lot of time with these people, and they will have a great deal of control over your working conditions. At one point in my career, I decided to move to sunny Florida and join a large multispecialty group with four other neurologists, with whom I could share call. It wasn't until I got there that I found out that this group was over $30 million in debt! When I quit, the group sued me for leaving, wanting all the salary and moving expenses they had paid me and for me to pay malpractice tail coverage as well. I moved on to join a solo practitioner I thought would be more ethical, only to find out that he had multiple physician assistants running rampant throughout the city unsupervised and doing some less than competent work. When I left that position, the physician sued me as well. These experiences left me with no other option but bankruptcy. I licked my wounds, moved back to Tennessee, and made the decision never to sign another contract with a large group again.

There is little control a physician employee can exert in a bad situation other than to move on. Because of that, the average physician these days will change jobs seven times during his or her career. This is a huge change from the past, when physicians were an integral part of a community and spent their entire careers in the same area. Now, as often as patients change insurance, physicians may find themselves moving from state to state, looking for greener pastures that are, for the most part, no longer available. Many physicians are opting for temporary or locum tenens assignments, which involve working in various locations to fill in for vacationing physicians or for a group that is recruiting a permanent physician. The benefits to locum tenens include paid malpractice and travel expenses without any overhead, good pay with incentives for being on call, and a chance to check out a region the physician may be interested in, while no permanent commitment is required. The drawback is the traveling and having to be away from family and friends for extended periods of time. There is no chance to bond with the patients in long-term relationships. In addition, there can be a lot of downtime in between jobs and no paid health insurance or other benefits. I decided to try locum tenens work instead of signing any more long-term, restrictive contracts. The locum tenens work was fun, exciting, and challenging, as I had to adjust and learn new hospital computer systems and layouts and new office procedures, and meet all new patients on the fly. I did miss the long-term relationships with my patients and the sense of community I had in my small-town private practice of the past. I missed my family, as I was often displaced for months at a time. I tried to focus on what it was that gave me a sense of fulfillment from the practice of medicine. As I searched my soul, I concluded that I never should have left the sheltered halls of the university and that I should look for a teaching position, even though it meant a large pay cut. I did succeed in becoming an assistant professor, and I loved teaching medical students and residents in my new job, but it was no bed of roses. The politics of the university, the pressure to get research grants, and the necessity of dealing with a disorganized bureaucracy was very frustrating, especially after having had my own practice with a staff that catered to me. I was low man on the totem pole in the university and was continually reminded of that.

## INCREASING UNPAID TIME

In the past, the cost of caring for uninsured patients was absorbed in the practice with little difficulty, since most people had commercial insurance or Medicare that paid well enough to make up the difference. There was a range of payment amounts that included commercial insurance, Medicare, Medicaid, and the uninsured. The high-end payments compensated for the lack of reimbursement from the uninsured patients we saw each day. We didn't have to worry about HMOs or PPOs that affected the patients' copayments or coverage. Most physicians considered it their duty to care for a percentage of the indigent population. Most physicians agree that difficult circumstances shouldn't keep people from receiving health care even if they can't pay for it. However, now that there are more than fifty million people with no health insurance, physicians can no longer afford to take on the burden our society has created, where so many are left out in the cold and have to use the emergency room as their only source of medical attention, neglecting chronic illnesses until they are in dire straits. Politicians seem to feel that doctors and hospitals should continue to absorb the burden of America's uninsured population, which has become untenable. With the recent passage of the Patient Protection and Affordable Care Act, at least more patients will be covered, and physicians will be reimbursed something for more of the patients they see, even if it is less overall per patient (Patient Protection and Affordable Care Act, HR03590, 2010). However, most physicians are pessimistic about the way the proposed changes will affect them. The regulations and requirements that are meant to cut down on health care costs are likely to be prohibitive to small groups or solo physicians. The health insurance "Chinese menu" of benefits that physicians have to sort through with each individual patient is likely to get more complex, and the pressure to see more patients will likely increase. Reimbursement rates are likely to decrease further.

Because of the rising rates of uninsured or minimally insured people, medicine has become a multitiered caste system. We have to factor the patient's insurance type into every medical decision we make. For instance, if a patient has no insurance, they not only can't be seen in the office without paying cash up front, but they won't be able to afford any tests or treatments that the physician deems necessary. If they are hospitalized, we must attempt to get every test that we can done before discharge, putting the burden of that cost on the hospital. They won't be able to get these tests done in an outpatient setting without insurance or payment up front. If patients have no insurance, the medication we select for their conditions must be available in a generic form and cheap enough for them to afford it. This might be okay for common medical problems, but many times there are no cheap generic alternatives available. If the patient cannot afford the tests, medications, or treatments we recommend, how much can we help them? Are we supposed to turn a blind eye—as so many politicians in Washington have—to the suffering of our less wealthy, uninsured brothers and sisters?

Physicians may not be the best businessmen; we want to put our patients' health first, regardless of cost considerations. It is a sad fact that physicians have given up control of our field to the powerful insurance companies, pharmaceuticals, and the government. We have become pawns in the field of medicine to be controlled and pushed in directions that don't make U.S. health care the best—only the most expensive and administratively complicated. Small groups of people, CEOs, insurance executives, and administrative middlemen are walking away with millions or even billions of dollars that are desperately needed to keep our whole population healthy. They average thirty one percent of the health care dollar for administrative costs, versus about three percent for Medicare. Their goal is profit, not the health of the nation's people. They want their piece of the health care dollar. The U.S. spends nearly twice as much on health care as the other countries with national health plans, and have worse health outcomes and over 50 million uninsured. If we could get rid of the middlemen, there would just be doctors and patients, lower hospital and medication costs, and better-quality health care. To achieve such a goal, patients and doctors need to come together. We need to pressure our congressmen to stop listening to the powerful lobbyists of the insurance companies, managed care companies, the pharmaceutical companies and the trial lawyers.

The moral and ethical principles that physicians live by have been used against them time and time again. Insurance companies know that physicians will see patients when they are seriously ill, regardless of whether they will get paid. If a patient shows up with an emergency, doctors will try to help that individual, even if it means getting up at two am to drive in to the hospital. However, they may never get paid for what is often the most difficult part of their jobs. Frequent denials for payment after care has been delivered leave tens or hundreds of thousands of dollars' worth of services unpaid each year. It is common practice for many insurance companies routinely to deny payment for services when the first bill is submitted. This ends up taking up more of the physician's and his or her staff's time and disturbs the normal cash flow of the business. These denials frequently turn into paperwork nightmares, with physicians having to resubmit their charges over and over, with more documentation. Only after multiple submissions, with copies of the patient's records, does the insurance company finally pay some of these bills. That extra time required is not reimbursed by insurance companies or patients. It's no wonder that so many physicians have stopped taking ER call or seeing hospitalized patients.

Attorneys charge for every minute they spend working on a client's case, but physicians are only paid for the time they spend directly with the patient. They don't get paid for reviewing labs and test results, literature research, calling in prescriptions, calling the patient or speaking with family members, even though these activities take up a large portion of each day. They don't get paid for being on call, only for the patients they have seen face-to-face during that time. Answering phone calls or emails from patients, calling in prescriptions, or responding to pages from the hospital staff all night long are not reimbursable.

I found that in doing business, both professionally and personally, when people found out that I was a doctor, they assumed I could afford to pay top dollar for everything. The costs of medical supplies and equipment were artificially jacked up just because they were for medical use. Even as consumers in unrelated business dealings, we were often taken advantage of when we were identified as doctors. Many physicians avoided telling business associates that they are doctors, because that diminished their chances for negotiating a better deal.

The attitudes of our patients often seemed to be that doctors were all uniformly wealthy, charge too much, and could afford to lose money on their bills, while still supplying medical care whenever they were needed. Their medical bills may seem very high for the amount of time spent with them. Very few people have any insight into what goes on behind the scenes of a medical practice. That is why I hope to open people's eyes about the business issues that make practicing medicine today so difficult.

Overall, the business of running a medical practice is very complex and difficult. Frequent changes in the coding procedures and requirements of running a practice are making things even worse. If the new Health Care Act is fully enacted, the requirements of physicians are going to be so complex and costly, it will be nearly impossible for individual private-practice physicians to comply with all the regulations. The penalties for mistakes or noncompliance will be increased. Those physicians who have supplemented their income by ownership in other health care facilities, like hospitals or imaging centers will be penalized and ineligible for Medicare and Medicaid payments. Some physicians are opting for concierge practices, where patients pay them a monthly fee directly, and they have access to their physicians on an as-needed basis. The patients are expected to file paperwork to get reimbursed by their insurance companies. For those who cannot afford the concierge option, shortages of physicians will be exacerbated, as more patients seek care. More and more "physician extenders" like nurse practitioners and physician assistants will replace the rigorously trained physician. The liability for these personnel will still sit upon the physician's shoulders, however. In addition, the reimbursement is scheduled to continue decreasing, with no obligations on insurance companies to improve their payment processes to physicians. In a survey by Merritt Hawkins and Associates, most physicians plan to retire, work part-time, locum tenens, or as concierge physicians, which will further exacerbate the shortage of physicians (The Physicians Foundation, 2008). Seminars on nonclinical careers for physicians have become popular.

Even physicians who work for large groups or HMOs are feeling the pinch of reduced reimbursements and expenses as they are pushed to see more and more patients in less and less time. The moral and ethical considerations of providing medical care to all of those who need it are at odds with the need to run a successful business. More and more physicians find themselves refusing to treat those who are uninsured, or those who cannot pay for their medical care. They know that if they don't focus on every penny coming in and going out, they will be unable to treat any patients at all. Morale is reaching all-time lows among physicians, and unless something is done there will be no physician to show up in the ER at two AM for the next life-threatening emergency (Jacob, 2002).

Physicians have very little control over their income or expenses, as insurance companies and the government dictate their decreasing payment rates and malpractice and health insurance rates rise by double digits each year. The solo practitioners and small groups of physicians are closing their doors at alarming rates, physicians over fifty are retiring or plan to retire within the next three years, and job satisfaction is at an all-time low (Steiger, 2007). Even young residents graduating from training are questioning their careers before they even get started (Robert Wood Johnson Foundation, 2000). A full 24 percent stated they would choose a different career if they had their education to do over again. As physicians work harder and harder for lower and lower incomes, the incentive to sacrifice one's life for the noble career of healing is diminished. The stress of trying to practice medicine under these conditions affects the attitudes of physicians and potential physicians in all aspects of their lives.

# CHAPTER 4:
## LIABILITY IN MEDICINE

One of the hardest lessons of life in medicine is that of liability. Once we take on a patient as our own, we are liable for his or her health in ways that we never before dreamed. The very word *malpractice* strikes fear into the heart of most physicians. A single malpractice lawsuit can put an end to the career of a physician who spent half of his or her life preparing for it. It doesn't matter how great a physician you are; every time you see a patient, you are at risk. Every time you offer advice over the phone to a fellow physician or to a patient, you are at risk. Every time you write a prescription, you are at risk. Even if you do everything right in caring for a patient, a bad outcome puts you at risk. For the physician, the inner knowledge of our own imperfection is constantly at odds with the expectations of our patients to be perfect in diagnosis and treatment.

If people can understand how difficult it is to practice medicine, with all of its variables, with all of its demands, then how can they expect perfection in each individual case? Physicians are human beings. They cannot keep track of every detail of each day or of each patient. They cannot predict or prevent all possible complications from occurring. Mistakes will happen, unfortunately with some physicians more than others. However, it is extremely rare that willful negligence plays a role in most bad outcomes.

## MALPRACTICE CLAIMS ARE ON THE RISE

The incidence of malpractice cases has increased over recent years. In addition, the amounts of malpractice payments have also increased dramatically. The median medical malpractice payout was $99,500 in

2000, over $175,000 in 2006. The mean payouts were $202,301 in 2000 and $311,965 in 2006, according to the National Practitioner Data Bank, which includes all payments, including those that were settled out of court (National Practitioner Data Bank Annual Reports, 2000; 2006). In 2001, 5 percent of all payouts were over $1 million. In addition, in 2002, only 5 percent of all physicians were responsible for over 50 percent of all malpractice lawsuits. According to a Towers/Perrin Report, the total tort costs for medical malpractice in 1994 was $6.3 million, in 2007 $16.9 million (Watson, 2010).

Lawyers have played a large role in causing the escalation of health care costs. Malpractice claims have not only been increasing in number, but the amounts of jury awards have become extravagant, as well. The lawyers keep anywhere from 30 to 40 percent of a successful verdict awarded, and this can amount to millions for a single successful case they litigate. This has had a twofold effect on costs. The insurance companies raise their rates, and doctors practice defensive medicine. In a study published in 2005 in the Journal of the American Medical Association, 93 percent of physicians surveyed reported practicing defensive medicine (*Journal of the American Medical Association*, 2005). Insurance companies reported spending an average of $30 billion in defending and paying out legal expenses over the past several years (Steiger, 2007). Thirty billion dollars could go a long way toward providing everyone in this country with top-quality health care.

Documentation is supposedly the key to avoiding lawsuits, but I have found that honest communication with, and compassion for my patients are really the key. If a patient or his or her family seems unhappy or mistrustful of my diagnosis or opinion, I am quick to refer them for a second opinion if they want it. If an unexpected bad outcome occurs, immediate disclosure and discussion with the family is helpful. However, there are many people out there who are simply looking for an opportunity to sue a physician for personal reward and instant riches. It is a sad fact that most physicians now see each patient as a potential lawsuit, and rightfully so, since 7.4 percent of all physicians nationwide per year can expect to be sued. In states like Florida and Pennsylvania, this number is higher. A recent study by the New England Journal of Medicine reported that 75 per cent of physicians in low-risk specialties and 99 percent of physicians in high-risk specialties can expect to be sued for malpractice during their careers (Jena, 2011). For me, having never been sued in twelve years of practice was probably more a matter of luck than skill.

Lawyers are very good at playing Monday-morning quarterback, and by poring through medical records, they can often find some omission or undocumented factor that they can use to convince a jury that negligence or willful injury has occurred. Expert witnesses are paid by these lawyers to find something that can be used against the treating physician. The old cliché, "Hindsight is 20/20," has never been a more effective tool for lawyers and their expert witnesses. Though I have never been sued for malpractice (knock on wood), I am as paranoid about it as any of my colleagues who have been sued. Even if a physician manages to weather a lawsuit professionally and emotionally, the increase in overhead, particularly malpractice insurance, can end a physician's career. The recording of a malpractice judgment against a physician follows them throughout their careers and can prevent them from getting jobs, medical licenses, or hospital privileges in the future.

Even those physicians who have never been sued have been conditioned to look for red flags of potentially litigious patients. They are taught to stay on the defensive and never admit any mistake or guilt. They are taught that if it wasn't documented, it wasn't done. Yet it is impossible to document fully the entire visit with each patient unless we start making videos of every patient encounter.

In many places around the country, commercials, billboards, telephone books, and newspapers advertise legal firms that specialize in malpractice and proclaim the huge awards they have gotten for their clients. "Burt Dunham got me two million dollars!", claims a dancing lady. One advertisement on television in Florida goes, "If you have a loved one in a nursing home, call us." The ad doesn't even mention whether you felt some wrongdoing had taken place. Given the opportunity, a lawyer and his expert witnesses can find something that can be used to build a malpractice claim. Not all attorneys or expert witnesses are that unscrupulous.

People have to take more responsibility for their illnesses and accept that when illness strikes, there is often little that a doctor can do. People in nursing homes are generally there because they are close to death and unable to care for themselves. They have no family able or willing to care for them at home. A nursing home can never replace the individual home and family environment. It is not always the physician's or the nursing home staff's fault if Aunt Molly fell out of bed and broke her hip. Nursing home regulations strictly forbid the use of restraints in most patients even when they have been identified as being at-risk for falls, and their reimbursement rates have been cut down so far that they usually cannot afford to staff their facilities adequately. Running a nursing home in this day and age is very difficult, expensive, and overrun with administrative costs and paperwork. Running a hospital is also very tough, and liability issues are threatening to close more doors of small non-profit hospitals that cannot afford the rising insurance rates and incidence of lawsuits

There are many successful lawsuits based on poor outcomes or delay of diagnosis in patients with difficult diagnostic challenges in which there is no negligence, misconduct, or harmful intent by the physician. Lawyers and their clients must face the fact that people get sick and die every day, no matter what physicians do. Years of bad habits, illness, and the natural process of aging will take their toll, and while Americans often look to blame someone else for their misfortunes, physicians are tired of being the scapegoats.

# EXAMPLES OF SUCCESSFUL MALPRACTICE LAWSUITS

A pregnant woman presented to the ER at a teaching hospital with abdominal pain. The resident who saw her admitted her and determined that she had an abruption of the placenta—a separation of the lining of the placenta with bleeding internally. I am not an obstetrician, but I recall from my medical school days that this is one of the most feared complications of pregnancy, and it carries a high risk of mortality no matter what physicians do. It is difficult to diagnose and treat. The woman was in fact properly diagnosed in this case, and within one hour of arrival to the hospital, an emergency C-section was performed. However, the baby suffered severe brain damage from the loss of blood in the umbilical cord. It was a sad case with a bad outcome. Of course, a lawsuit was filed claiming that a forty-six minute delay in the treatment constituted negligence on the part of the physicians and caused the baby's brain damage. The lawsuit was successful and awarded $75 million to the parents for future costs of home care, another $13 million for the future cost of medical care, another $2 million for loss of earnings of the child, and $760,000 for pain and suffering. Had an obstetrician not been available, both mother and baby would probably have died.

One of my colleagues was sued by the sister of a young man with severe cerebral palsy and speech impediment. This patient was admitted to the hospital after falling out of his wheelchair. He had been born disabled and had always been wheelchair bound. He had continuous uncontrollable movements of his head, arms, and legs. He had poor communication skills because of severe speech impediments. There was very little that he could do for himself. His sister said that he had fallen out of his wheelchair and lost some additional use of his arms. My friend saw him and appropriately ordered an MRI of his cervical spine to check for a herniated disc. Unfortunately, the patient moved too much for the MRI scan to be completed. A second MRI was ordered the following day, with sedation. Again the patient's movements interfered with a successful scan. The weekend arrived, and I was on call, covering for my friend. When I went to see this patient, he had been moved to rehabilitation for further treatment, and a third attempt at an MRI failed, again because of the patient's excess movement. I ordered a CT myelogram, a more invasive test that involves putting dye into the spinal canal and then performing a CT scan. It is a less sensitive test than the MRI, and exposes the patient to radiation, but one in which some movement can be tolerated. I insisted on the radiologist coming in on a Sunday evening to perform the test, and it showed a large herniated disc in the patient's neck. The patient went to surgery the next day, and his herniated disc was successfully treated. Later on, the true history was revealed about how the family attempted to get him up after his fall by dragging him by the arm, which probably caused the disc to rupture. Over the next few months he improved and returned to his baseline. However, his sister sued the hospital, the primary care doctor, and my neurology colleague for "delay in diagnosis," claiming that it caused the young man to become more disabled. Because of his uncontrolled movements and because the family withheld part of the history about the details of his fall, it took a week to diagnose the herniated disc. This was a young man who was severely disabled since birth, and it was difficult for these physicians who had never seen him before to differentiate a new deficit from the old deficits with which he was born.

I remember well when the lawyers came and took my deposition. A confident, well-dressed young attorney waltzed into my office with his entourage of assistants and a court reporter. I was a bit nervous and expressed my concern about testifying in this case. I had only covered a weekend. The lawyer said, "Relax, we're not suing you. You're the 'hero' in this case." Wow! If ever such a title was less welcome … I was amazed and appalled at the craftiness with which he constructed his questions, leading me down a path of pity for the innocent victim and outrage toward the terrible doctors and therapists who I knew had taken very good care of this severely disabled, highly complicated patient. I felt like an unwilling Brutus. My friend and colleague is a brilliant neurologist, an MD/PhD. He was also one of the most intelligent, devoted, and loved physicians in his community. He didn't do anything wrong, and negligence had nothing to do with the difficulties this patient encountered.

After surgery this patient actually returned to his baseline of severe disability with slightly more voluntary arm movement. It came to light during the trial that the sister had once worked for the hospital and had been fired. Her grudge against the hospital was never recognized as a motive for suing the hospital and the doctors involved in her brother's care. Despite all these complicated factors, her lawyers succeeded in getting a 1.2 million-dollar settlement for the young man's sister to spend as she saw fit. He continued to get all his medical care paid for by Medicare and Medicaid as he had throughout his lifetime.

How do you think this malpractice lawsuit affected my friend? Every time a physician is sued, it's like cutting the legs out from under them. We have to get out on the tightrope again, every day. We must try to balance the life-and-death issues we are faced with and take chances on making mistakes as we do our best to help people in crisis. When a physician holds the scalpel in his hand, it must be steady and confident, not trembling and insecure. Do you realize that a physician will never see his patients or his career in the same way after experiencing a lawsuit? Fortunately, my friend kept practicing, although he moved to another state where the incidence of malpractice lawsuits is lower. Another friend of mine was not so lucky.

There was a nineteen-year-old girl with epilepsy. Her seizures were well controlled and she had been awarded a driver's license. Based on a decision by the Department of Motor Vehicles, in most states driver's licenses are awarded to epileptic patients whose seizures have been well controlled for a year on medication. In California, my friend was required to file a form with the Department of Motor Vehicles reporting the young woman as a seizure patient.

At one point, she had a breakthrough seizure. Her medications were adjusted, and the neurologist told her not to drive again until they could tell whether the medication changes were successfully preventing her seizures. There was no requirement to file another form with the DMV; at some point you have to rely on patients to be compliant and to take responsibility for their own behavior. However, this patient did not listen to her doctor, and while driving around with one of her friends, she had a seizure and crashed the car. Both girls survived, but the friend broke her neck and became quadriplegic. Her lawyers sued everyone they could, including the neurologist. Because the epileptic girl's family had no money and limited insurance, the jury found my friend guilty of malpractice because he didn't send a *second* form to the DMV at the time he told her not to drive. Re-filing forms with the DMV every time we see an epileptic patient is not a requirement. Yet, somehow he was guilty of not predicting that this patient would disobey his verbal instructions not to drive. Somehow filing a second form would have prevented that accident from happening. They won their case for $3 million. Although the neurologist was determined to have only 5 percent liability in this case, his was the "deep pocket"; he was expected to pay the entire amount, and he lost practically everything he had. Deep pockets means that in cases where multiple defendants were sued, the individuals with the money or insurance to pay have to shoulder the entire cost, even if they were found to have a small percentage of liability in a case. After twenty years of service to this community in California, he closed his doors and walked away. It was a devastating blow to his spirit as well as to his career. In a broader sense, this Harvard-trained physician of incredible skill and great respect was lost to all his thousands of patients, both present and future, because of this one lawsuit.

Another case describes a woman who injured her heel stomping on aluminum cans. She continued to walk on the foot for two weeks before seeking any medical attention. The primary care physician she saw ordered an X-ray, which showed an old fracture. He ordered a rheumatology consult since she continued to have pain, and then an orthopedic surgery consult. Unfortunately there was damage done from her bearing weight on the foot the entire time, and surgery on the heel was complicated, leading to a partial amputation of the heel. She successfully sued the primary care physician for not putting her on non-weight-bearing status when he saw her, even though she admitted to walking on the heel for two weeks before she even saw a doctor for the problem. She was awarded $1.45 million.

Another case was that of a middle-aged man who had neck pain and a ruptured disc. His doctor ordered the appropriate tests and diagnosed his neck condition. Some blood tests were also ordered at the initial visit. The patient did not show up for his return appointment to go over the blood tests but did get a referral to a specialist, who operated on his neck. Later on, several months after the surgery, the patient returned to his doctor, who informed him of a low vitamin $B_{12}$ level that showed up in his blood tests from the prior visit. The patient sued the doctor for failing to notify him of the $B_{12}$ deficiency and was awarded millions of dollars. The main problem, the large disc herniation in his neck, had been successfully treated. If the patient had shown up for his follow-up appointment, he would have found out about the $B_{12}$ deficiency at that time. Again, no permanent damage was sustained, and because doctors have thousands of patients to see each year, they simply cannot possibly keep track of all the results in all patients at all times, especially when they don't show up for their follow-up visits. When patients miss appointments, the physician cannot be expected to track them down. Patients must take some responsibility for their own health, and if they have not been informed of a test result, they should call their doctor's offices to get those results. No matter how efficiently a doctor's office is run, test results can slip through the cracks. Is failure to notify a no-show patient of an abnormal test result reason enough for a million-dollar lawsuit?

Another case involved a man in his fifties with long-standing, untreated hypertension. He showed up at the hospital complaining of dizziness. His blood pressure was treated, and he was given a prescription for the blood pressure. A few hours after he went home, the dizziness got worse, and he returned to the ER and was admitted. During the night, he had a massive stroke in the back of his brain. When his symptoms worsened, a neurology consult was requested. The neurologist determined through an exam that the patient's brain had been irreparably damaged. Because of the severity of his stroke, he was diagnosed as brain dead and would be unable to recover. The family sued the hospital, the ER physician, and the neurologist for not transferring him to another hospital for a neurosurgery consult, which they claimed would have saved his life. However, most neurologists know that in a case like this, the odds of survival are minuscule, and if he had survived, he would most likely have spent his last days as a vegetable. Had he controlled his blood pressure with medication, this complication could have been prevented. Strokes are the third leading cause of death in our country, and our ability to predict or prevent them is limited and mostly based on lifestyle changes for which the patient is responsible. The most important prevention is to treat risk factors like hypertension.

These cases all have something in common. The patient in each case had a bad outcome. They all had complications of their underlying illness. The lawyers claimed that the doctors should have been able to predict and prevent the complications that occurred. However, physicians are not only unable to predict bad outcomes, but they are often helpless to prevent or even treat them.

It would be great if physicians were capable of perfection in their diagnoses and treatments, had 100 percent efficiency in their offices, and kept track of every patient they saw as if they were the only patient they had. It would be great if we could control our patients' behaviors and compliance with our treatment plans. It would be great if we were psychic and could predict the future for our patients and our treatments. Unfortunately, these lofty goals can never be reached. If we are liable for not being perfect, then we should all be sued and just give up trying to practice medicine. There are great doctors, but not one of them is perfect. Many of the best doctors have had the most lawsuits filed against them. This is especially true of professors in university hospitals who oversee the care of many indigent patients who show up in the emergency room in crisis and have more bad outcomes. Some of the worst doctors have never been sued. Many legitimate cases of negligence never make it to the courts. The medico-legal system is not weeding out the bad doctors or improving medical care in America. Being sued certainly does not improve a doctor's skills or reform him or her into being a better doctor. It's all about the money.

With very few exceptions, most of the lawsuits I have heard about are similar to these cases. They involve poor outcomes with pitiful "victims." Deeply flawed logic is dressed up in a tragic drama portrayed by skilled lawyers. They enact a scenario portraying doctors as evil or incompetent and patients as innocent victims, a picture that is often far removed from reality. There is no regard for the ripple effects that cases like these have. It's all about the money.

## CONSEQUENCES OF MALPRACTICE LITIGATION

Every time a lawsuit is filed, there are far-reaching consequences for health care. Malpractice insurance rates for doctors and hospitals have risen dramatically (Albert, 2003). There have been dramatic increases in the rates every year for the past several years, raising the cost of practice overhead. Doctors and hospitals cut back on high-risk procedures that increase their rates, and this hurts the sickest patients most of all. Doctors practice defensive medicine, ordering extra tests and procedures that may be unnecessary, just to be all-inclusive of the differential diagnosis of a given symptom, and this raises the costs of health care and health insurance dramatically. Doctors quit practicing medicine or move to other states that have lower incidences of malpractice lawsuits or laws that limit malpractice awards. They stop seeing ER patients or hospitalized patients at all. They stop doing high-risk procedures even if they may be life-saving. Since doctors have to work that much harder to cover their malpractice premiums, they see more patients in less time and the doctor-patient relationship suffers. In the end, doctors and patients both pay the price while attorneys cash in.

The expectations of perfection by lawyers, injured patients, and sympathetic juries have led to many huge jury awards. Of all the malpractice cases awarded each year, very few are truly documented cases of malpractice. In fact, 80 percent of all malpractice lawsuits filed have been dropped, dismissed, or found in favor of the physician. Sixty percent of these lawsuits are considered to be without merit and are dropped or dismissed. Many cases, however, are settled by insurance companies—often against the wishes of the physician—out of fear of unpredictable juries sympathetic to patients with poor outcomes. Approximately 1 percent of all malpractice lawsuits filed result in successful verdicts for the plaintiffs, and, as you can see from the above examples, many of these are questionable in terms of physician guilt or negligence (Stuudert, 2006). A recent report from the American Medical Association shows that there are 95 claims per 100 doctors per year, in this country—nearly one per physician. The numbers in the high-risk specialties like neurosurgery, obstetrics, and general surgery are staggering (Todd, 2010).

Advertising by lawyers has reached a feverish pitch as well, especially in places like Florida. The commercials on TV and radio and in the phone books are more and more unethical, promising riches to those who call, whether they think they have a case or not. Meanwhile, state governments are controlled by lawyers in politics, who have put up a wall blocking any meaningful tort reform. Tort reform would place monetary limits on the amounts of malpractice awards for pain and suffering, although not on the actual costs of health care incurred or future health care needs. Because of the rising incidence of lawsuits, many insurance companies have pulled out of states like Florida and no longer issue policies for malpractice insurance. Of course, the rates of those insurers still in Florida have skyrocketed with the increased demand for coverage (Florida Medical Malpractice Insurance History, 2000–2010). There are no punitive damages for frivolous lawsuits filed by unscrupulous lawyers, which cost physicians and their insurance companies tens of thousands of dollars to defend, even when they are dismissed. However, in Texas, a loser-pays rule has cut down significantly on frivolous lawsuits. This means that legal costs incurred by the defense are paid by the prosecution.

When I started out in practice in the early nineties, my malpractice liability insurance rates were about $1,200 per year. In Tennessee, in 2001, my annual rate was $5,200. However, I moved to Florida, and the rate there was $12,000 per year in 2001. Despite my having a perfectly clean record, with no claims or complaints against me, the rate in 2003 would have been $35,000 per year to renew, for one-fourth of the coverage I had previously. I could not afford that, as well as the increasing overhead in Florida, so I left, breaking my contract, and moved back to Tennessee. Similar conditions are being experienced by physicians in many states across the country, such as Pennsylvania, North Carolina, and Nevada, where an exodus of physicians is directly due to malpractice claims and the cost of malpractice insurance (Hellinger, 2002). Although I had never been sued in eleven years of practicing, I was expected to pay more than six times the rates I had paid just two years earlier. Neurologists don't make that much money compared to other specialists; we take more time with our patients and we perform few high-dollar procedures. Most neurologists simply cannot afford the insurance rates they are expected to pay nowadays, and more and more are simply unwilling to work even harder just to line the pockets of insurance companies and lawyers.

Obstetricians have seen their malpractice insurance rates increase ten times or more from what it was ten years ago, and all specialties have seen the options for shopping or comparing rates go down, because many insurers are pulling out of these "high-risk" states. Many have quit the practice of obstetrics, no longer delivering babies because of the risk of lawsuits related to poor outcomes and the cost of malpractice insurance (Merritt Hawkins and Associates Summary Report, 2003). There are many counties in Florida where there are no obstetricians available and pregnant women have to travel hours to get prenatal care and to have their babies. Just imagine, going into labor and having a three-hour ride in the car to get to your doctor! Even worse, what if there is a complication and you end up in the local ER? One of the most natural processes that women go through—a typically joyful, uncomplicated experience—has been tainted by the legal and insurance businesses, which have driven good doctors from their own communities and made it difficult for everyone to obtain safe, quality care. Caring for patients in states like Pennsylvania with high malpractice insurance rates has led physicians to report rising job dissatisfaction and reduced quality of care (Mello, 2004).The situation is only getting worse, and by the time people wake up and realize that there is a huge shortage of physicians, it will be too late for this sue-crazy generation.

Many physicians in Florida are going "bare," carrying no malpractice insurance, placing a sign in their offices advising patients of their decision to keep their doors open the only way that they can. They have patients read the statement and sign a waiver not to sue the doctor if they are seen and treated. These physicians cannot get hospital privileges without malpractice insurance because the bylaws of most hospitals require it, so they can only practice outpatient medicine. Many insurance companies will not allow an uninsured physician be a provider. These physicians often practice on a cash basis, and the patients are expected to send their bill to the insurance company and fight with them for payment. These doctors are literally trying to practice medicine with one hand tied behind their backs. They are still at risk of being sued, despite their warnings to patients; however, when the pot of gold over their heads (insurance payout) is gone, many lawyers are unwilling to take on these cases, so these doctors are often left alone. These physicians take their chances and protect their assets as best they can. Certain assets cannot be taken in the event of a verdict against the physician, such as their homes, life insurance policies, and retirement funds. However, there is a significant risk that a physician could end up in bankruptcy and lose any other savings or assets he or she has in the event of a malpractice lawsuit.

Physicians are also put in the awkward situation of being liable for the patient's complications if a test that was not done initially shows a significant problem that could have been treated more successfully if caught earlier, like a tumor. We can also be considered liable if a medication or treatment that was denied by insurance would have prevented worsening of the patient's condition. If an insurance company denies approval for a test or treatment in this situation, the doctor can be liable if they don't fight for approval on the patient's behalf and help the patient find some alternative.

People used to complain that their doctors acted as if they were gods. Nowadays, people expect their doctors to *be* gods—perfect in their diagnoses and treatments, and even able to predict the future. They expect physicians to cure all diseases and prevent death, even though it is the inevitable process we all go through at some point in our lives. The reality is that there are very few true cures in medicine. Physicians are able to help patients delay death in a small percentage of cases and only temporarily. Our medicines, surgeries, and other treatments are far from perfect and are fraught with potential side effects and complications. In a given study, there may be a 10 percent chance of a side effect to a medication, but if your patient is the one who develops that side effect, it doesn't matter what percentage they're in. They are not going to be happy with you, and if the situation is life-threatening or has a bad outcome, there is a pretty good chance they will sue.

When a bad outcome occurs for a patient under treatment by a physician, the patient and their family often look for someone to blame. America has become a blame-oriented, lawyer-crazy society, and this problem extends beyond the field of medicine. Physicians, being human, will inevitably fail to live up to the expectations of perfection in the battle against death. The people on these juries often feel sorry for the injured parties, but there isn't always a connection to negligence on the part of the physicians.

Medical mistakes were reported to have caused serious complications or death in 44,000 to 98,000 people in one year (Institute of Medicine Committee on Quality of Health Care in America, 2000). This meant all medical errors, not just those of physicians, and included medication errors on the parts of hospitals, pharmacies, and nurses, for example. This seems like a lot of mistakes, but it is taken out of context. This number is, in fact, a small percentage of the millions of patient encounters that occur in one year. Lawyers try to increase their odds of winning a verdict by suing everyone involved in the patient's care, from the hospital to each and every physician involved in the care of the patient. It's no wonder the numbers of malpractice claims and the amounts of awards increase each year. It's also no wonder that trial lawyers are some of the highest-paid professionals in this country and have such control of politics, blocking legislation to control and cap malpractice awards. Tort costs in 2001 were over $200 billion, with an estimated income for trial lawyers of over $40 billion (Copland, 2003). Given that most politicians are lawyers, one can see the tremendous power this group has in blocking tort reform that would cut into lawyers' pocketbooks significantly.

In recent years, however, there has been some progress in passing legislation that helps physicians by placing a cap on the amount of noneconomic damages (for pain and suffering, not for the actual medical costs or lost wages) a jury can award to a family in the case of a poor outcome due to physician negligence or malpractice. Twenty-six states now have similar laws to prevent those jackpot jury awards that are so enticing to patients and their lawyers. Malpractice insurance rates have improved in these states, and physicians are no longer leaving these areas in large numbers. No conclusive studies have shown that these laws actually help improve the quality of patient care or prevent malpractice from occurring, however. Physicians all over the country are still gun-shy about malpractice liability.

People justify suing their doctors and hospitals by saying, "Oh, this should teach that doctor a lesson," or "He deserves to pay for his mistakes." If every doctor was forced to pay for all their mistakes, they wouldn't bother to try. Every time we accept a new patient as our own, write a prescription, perform a procedure, mistakes occur either by commission or omission. We just don't let our fear of failure keep us from trying to help others. If one of us makes a serious mistake, how is the transfer of millions of dollars going to teach us to do better? Physicians who are clearly negligent should go through additional training or have their licenses limited with some requirement for further supervision. These judgments should be carried out by medical professionals, and decisions regarding their ability to continue practice should be made by their peers, not lawyers, and not medically naive juries.

Physicians should be able to disclose a medical error without the risk of having that disclosure or an apology to the patient or family used against them in court. The error should be used as a teaching tool to help analyze the cause of the error and for prevention of future errors. A centralized compensation fund would reimburse patients for negligent medical errors in a no-fault system like those in New Zealand or Denmark, to help offset the costs, pain, and suffering involved in a poor outcome (Tanner, 2008). If physicians did not have to fear malpractice so much, they would be freer to report medical errors, police themselves better, and document a physician's performance that needed correcting (White et al., 2008). However, in our current system, documentation of hospital staff performance reviews or occurrences of medical errors can end up in a lawyer's hands. This can be a powerful weapon against a physician in court. A simple heartfelt apology from a physician to a patient who has suffered an unexpected or poor outcome can be considered an admission of guilt in a court of law.

Everyone knows that there are good, bad, and in between doctors out there. Physicians may be of a certain breed, but there is still a lot of variety among them. There are certainly some doctors who are truly negligent or willfully unethical. However, these are really a small minority of the thousands who have been sued successfully. It must be a tremendous temptation to sue a doctor who was in a hurry or who didn't seem sympathetic enough. If the doctor truly made a mistake that injured you or a loved one, this adds to the rationale for suing for as much as you can get.

The trial lawyers promise a potential jackpot of money that could turn most anyone's head. Then most people think, "What the heck, it's the insurance company's money, anyway, right? They've got plenty. The doctor isn't really going to lose anything, after all." Few people realize how a lawsuit can cut a physician to the bone. They don't realize that a single lawsuit can make a physician quit practicing medicine, or at the least change his or her perspective on this noble profession forever.

Increased malpractice insurance rates are passed on to patients by pharmaceutical companies, laboratories, HMOs, and hospitals, but cannot be adjusted by doctors, who are paid whatever the health insurance companies decide to pay. Obstetrics/gynecology is one of the specialties that has been hit the hardest with lawsuits, and physicians in this specialty have seen the highest malpractice insurance rate increases. Despite the fact that infant mortality has dropped 20 percent in the last ten years, obstetricians are one of the biggest targets of malpractice lawsuits for poor outcomes related to childbirth. Their medical liability insurance rates are on average in the six figures annually and continue to rise.

Malpractice lawsuits have far-reaching consequences that affect us all. The rapidly rising malpractice insurance rates are driving physicians out of certain states or out of practice at alarming rates. Many physicians have stopped doing high-risk procedures, cut back on emergency room coverage or gone part-time to reduce their insurance rates. This is already having a serious effect on access to medical care (Slepian, Lauren, 2003). Physicians have little choice but to restrict their practices in some way or to quit practicing altogether. Those physicians who stay in practice must increase their workload to make the premium payments. Inevitably, along with the increasing quantity of work, comes decreasing quality.

Many physicians have stopped taking ER call or doing any hospital care because it puts them at higher risk of lawsuits. Unfortunately, it is often the patients who show up in the ER at two AM who have no insurance coverage and who are most likely to sue the physicians who treat them. This may sound like a prejudicial statement, but most physicians and statistics will tell you that ER patients carry the highest liability risks and lowest reimbursement rates. They are the biggest source of stress and loss of sleep. Many physicians have stopped taking ER call for these reasons, leaving many emergency rooms without specialist coverage. This leaves the sickest patients without access to specialists in their greatest time of need.

Stroke, for example, is the third leading cause of death in America. It has also been the main source of litigation for neurologists in recent years. While this condition is devastating for those who succumb to it, there is very little that can be done to treat strokes once they occur, except for supportive care and rehabilitation. Although we have also made strides in stroke prevention, a cure or complete prevention is still out of reach. Sometimes the symptoms of stroke are difficult to diagnose, as they vary greatly, depending on the area of brain tissue affected, and can be missed initially, even by a trained neurologist. Once brain tissue has been damaged by a stroke, there is only a small window of a few hours, after which there is nothing a neurologist can do to bring that tissue back to life. Most strokes are due to the accumulation of atherosclerosis or "hardening of the arteries" over many years. Often the process is accelerated by bad dietary habits, smoking, or poor control of risk factors like hypertension, heart disease, and diabetes. As I described earlier, a treatment for acute stroke has become available, but it must be given within three hours of the onset of symptoms. It does not cure most strokes but improves the outcome over the next several months, leading to a better overall result. It has a potential side effect of causing bleeding and worsening of the stroke or even death. Of course, neurologists have to act fast in deciding whether a patient should receive this treatment and take the risk of a complication. This treatment has been a huge source of lawsuits for both giving the drug with complications and for not giving this drug to stroke patients in the ER. Lawyers often paint a picture that vilifies neurologists for failing to prevent or cure strokes, and when a sympathetic jury is persuaded to feel sorry for a patient injured by stroke, their reaction is to award money. By refusing to see patients in the hospital, neurologists can reduce their liability risks from stroke patients and their families, and their malpractice insurance rates go down. Some physicians have chosen this route to cut off the risk and the added stress of caring for hospitalized patients. Although this may be good for business, it is bad for health care and goes against the ethical principles physicians are expected to practice by.

Obstetrician/gynecologists are trained to deliver babies. Pregnancy is not a disease, it is a natural condition, and most of the time is associated with a great outcome for both mother and baby. The emotional and spiritual rewards of delivering babies are a primary reason most Ob/Gyn physicians choose this career. However, there are a small percentage of mothers and babies who have complications during delivery. Some mothers and babies will die, and some babies will have serious brain damage during the birthing process, and there is nothing anyone can do about it. However, the malpractice climate that has centered around complicated births has gone so far out of control, many Ob/Gyn physicians have stopped their obstetrical practices altogether. Because of defensive medicine, there are more Cesarean sections performed each year that may have been unnecessary. It is very difficult to get obstetrical care in many parts of the country, and the waiting time is often too long.

There is already a serious shortage of obstetricians in this country, particularly in states like Florida, Pennsylvania, and Illinois, where malpractice insurance rates and lawsuits are out of control. Some patients reserve their first prenatal appointments with the few remaining obstetricians in their communities before they even get pregnant, because of the long waiting periods to get in. Many women in America have no prenatal care and simply show up in the ER when they are in labor. Again, this often leads to more complications and more lawsuits. Midwives still have affordable insurance rates and have obstetricians as backups. If something goes wrong during delivery, the lawyers go after the backup physicians anyway, since they have the "deep pockets." This is called the "rule of joint and severable liability" in lawyer-speak. It says that all defendants are responsible for the full amount of an award regardless of the percentage of their fault or liability that was determined. For example, a patient has a car accident and suffers a complication of treatment in the hospital. The patient will typically sue the other driver, the car company, all the doctors who treated him or her, the hospital, and the makers of the treatment, whether that is a pharmaceutical company or an equipment manufacturer, etc. The jury may find the doctor 5 percent liable, but if the physician has more insurance or money than the others named in the lawsuit, he or she has to pay 100 percent, because he or she has the "deep pockets." Because of this, some physicians feel that they are less of a target when they don't carry large amounts of—or even any—malpractice insurance. The collateral source rule allows payment of the costs of medical care to be made even if the care was paid for by another source, such as health insurance. It doesn't mean that the patient has to pay the insurance company back; they just get a bonus of the money that was paid for their health care. Reforms of these regulations are part of the tort reform movement and in those states that have enacted reforms, malpractice insurance is going down (Hellinger et al., 2009).

The cost for a physician to defend against a claim is also a shock. Frivolous lawsuits that are dismissed or dropped amount to 61 percent of all malpractice cases that are filed and cost an average of $17,000 in legal expenses. The cases that actually go to trial and are successfully defended, cost an average of $86,000. Only one in seven cases that go to trial are decided in favor of the plaintiffs, and many of those are still questionable cases of malpractice, as the cases mentioned earlier will attest. Even if a frivolous case is brought against a physician, it goes on his or her record. The physician can be sure that his or her malpractice rates will be increased; or worse, he or she may be unable to get insurance at all. In states like Nevada and New Jersey, the major malpractice insurance providers stopped writing policies and left 50–60 percent of physicians scrambling to find alternative coverage or to move their practices to other states.

In 2001 physicians paid over $21 billion for malpractice insurance. This amount has doubled in the past ten years. Certain specialties like internal medicine, obstetrics/gynecology, neurosurgery, and general surgery have seen the biggest rises in rates.

As I have indicated, the malpractice insurance rates vary dramatically as well from state to state. In California, where tort reform has been in place for many years, an obstetrician may pay $13,000 per year, whereas in southern Florida the rates for the same physician with a clean record are over $200,000 (Lowes, 2010). The risk of being sued also varies from state to state, causing physicians to flee certain states toward low-risk areas and lower insurance rates. Are the doctors so much worse in some states that they deserve to be sued more often? This would seem pretty unlikely, considering that training and certification standards of medical practice are established on a nationwide basis. Perhaps it has more to do with the mentality of the citizens of some states and the legal profession's advertising habits that raises the likelihood of a lawsuit. The general attitude in this country of seeking to blame others every time an unexpected complication or bad outcome occurs may be more prevalent in certain cultures and regions within the country, which is the reason insurers raise rates in those areas.

The insurance companies claimed that in 2001 they paid out $1.34 for every $1.00 they collected in premiums. Studies have shown that this simply was not true. In many areas of the country, like southern Florida, many physicians simply could not purchase malpractice insurance at any price, especially if they had any prior claims on their records. The number of insurance companies offering malpractice insurance has also decreased dramatically. There were only a few companies in the Florida liability insurance market, which left price controls or competition by the wayside. However, recent studies have shown that there is little correlation between the cost of malpractice insurance and the number of claims paid out or actual losses, but that the cost is more related to competition between insurers and market dynamics. Exorbitant increases in malpractice insurance from 2000 to 2006 were unrelated to payouts, which actually decreased over that time period. When interest rates drop, or the stock market falls, insurance companies have less money to invest. They respond by increasing premiums and reducing coverage wherever they can. Profitability is the only goal for the vast insurance industry that controls nearly every aspect of a physician's practice (Americans for Insurance Reform, 2007).

## DEFENSIVE MEDICINE

The malpractice environment has changed the way physicians practice medicine. It is called defensive medicine. What is defensive medicine and why is it bad? Defensive medicine is defined as making treatment decisions based on avoiding lawsuits rather than the best interests of the patients. When patients visit their doctors, they bring a set of symptoms that are often vague and nonspecific, like dizziness, headache, or abdominal pain. It is often difficult to narrow the symptoms down to a single diagnosis. Part of our training as physicians is to take this set of symptoms and by asking specific questions, define and localize the symptoms further. The physical exam adds to the specificity and leads to a shorter list of possibilities, based on the patient characteristics and the statistical likelihood of certain diseases. Tests are ordered to confirm a diagnosis or to image a location where the symptoms or exam findings suggest an abnormality. Tests, whether blood or imaging, are generally expensive. If a disease is very rare and unlikely to be causing the symptoms, then it is not cost effective to order tests for that disease. However, if one in a thousand patients with a certain set of symptoms may have a rare condition, especially a life-threatening condition, then missing that one diagnosis could lead to a lawsuit that could end a physician's career. Physicians are pressured by managed care—and even receive financial incentives—to keep costs down. Yet if a diagnosis is missed, however unlikely it may have been, the physician, not the managed care organization, is the one placed in the defendant's seat. In fact, most managed care health insurance contracts have neat little clauses protecting them from lawsuits, which the patients must sign in order to get insurance coverage.

Headaches are one of the most common symptoms for which patients come to their doctor. The most common cause of headaches is migraine, a benign condition that is diagnosed by history and examination only. The chance that a patient with headaches has a brain tumor or an aneurysm is exceedingly small. However, with the fear of lawsuits in mind, more and more patients with the classical symptoms of migraine and normal examinations are being sent for MRI scans of the brain to rule out the one in a thousand chance that there is a tumor or aneurysm. With approximately 80 percent of the country having headaches, and the cost of MRI being about $2,000, the cost of obtaining MRI scans on all headache patients could run in the billions of dollars. Similarly, imagine that every patient with a chest cold gets a CT of the chest to rule out dissection of the aorta, or every patient with indigestion gets endoscopy or exploratory surgery to rule out ulcers or stomach cancer. Sometimes, a physician feels pressured into running tests he or she is certain will be normal because the patient has searched the Internet and read up on all the rare causes of his or her symptoms. The patient does not trust in the physician's experience and insists on getting the tests. If a physician refuses to do a test that a patient wants, this can be a setup for a lawsuit. In addition, patients will often go elsewhere until they find a physician who will run the test they want even if an abnormality is unlikely. With the time constraints on physicians' visits, there is often little time to fully examine a patient or to explain why they don't need a certain test. It is easier and safer from a defensive medicine standpoint to order the test and run up the costs of health care unnecessarily. These unnecessary tests may save a physician from a lawsuit, but they don't help the patient with his or her symptoms, and it can raise the level of anxiety about the possibility of a serious, undiagnosed medical condition. Physicians who have been burned by a missed diagnosis can develop a crisis of confidence in their abilities to diagnose a patient properly without the additional tests.

Studies have shown that the best way for a physician to avoid a lawsuit is to communicate effectively and sincerely with a patient and his or her family, particularly when a bad outcome occurs. Sometimes physicians taking care of the same patient don't even communicate well with each other to coordinate their care. Especially when a bad outcome occurs, they want to avoid being blamed or taking responsibility. I had a patient—we'll call him Mr. Williams—who passed out while he was out on the golf course. He was brought in to the hospital and initially was thought to have some type of cardiac problem. After that was ruled out, an EEG or brain-wave test was done, which showed epileptic activity and, with the history of confusion following his spell, I determined that he had actually had a seizure while golfing. I was consulted to see the patient, and as part of the workup, a MRI of his brain was done, and it showed a large aneurysm that was very likely to rupture and cause his death, if not treated. The neurosurgeon felt an operation was too risky because of the aneurysm's size, but a neuroradiologist felt that he could put a coil inside the aneurysm, and this would clot off the aneurysm sac and prevent rupture. There is a pretty high success rate with this type of procedure, and it is done through a catheter which is threaded through the groin into the brain, so no surgery is necessary. The patient would have to be put under anesthesia, however, so that they wouldn't move while this delicate procedure is being done. After a lengthy discussion of the risks and benefits with the patient and his family, they consented to have this procedure done.

On the scheduled day of the procedure, I waited to hear from the neuroradiologist about how things went, but no call came. The patient was delivered to the intensive care unit after the procedure, but no call from the nurses came. Finally, that evening, I stopped by the ICU and found my patient on a ventilator (breathing machine), and barely responsive. I gently shook him and then more vigorously tried to rouse him. I performed a more detailed neurological examination, finding no focal signs to suggest a stroke. It was a shock, yet no one seemed to know what had happened or when. I called the neuroradiologist, who said that, although the procedure had taken longer than expected, the coiling was successful. He did not know why the patient was not awake and alert. I did a CT scan to make sure there had been no bleeding, and the scan looked essentially normal. After I studied the operative records, it became apparent that the patient's blood pressure had dropped several times and was very unstable throughout the procedure. There had been prolonged periods of hypotension during the procedure that had not been corrected or controlled by the anesthesiologists. In addition, hypothermia or low body temperature, which can affect the body's autoregulation of heart rate, blood pressure, and many critical enzymes, had been significant during the procedure. Several different anesthesiologists had been in and out of the room taking turns monitoring the patient, since it had been a relatively long case, so no one had recognized that there was a problem when the patient failed to wake up normally afterward. They just dropped him off in the ICU on the ventilator when the procedure was completed, and seemed to have forgotten about him. There were no follow-up notes or explanations of why Mr. Williams was now in a coma. No one had bothered to inform me, as the attending physician, that there was any problem or that the patient had failed to return to his baseline, which was normal. When I contacted one of the anesthesiologists on the case, he became quite defensive and insisted that the problem must be due to the coiling procedure, not any fault of the anesthesiologists or the repeated and prolonged blood pressure and temperature drops that had occurred during the procedure. I am a neurologist, yet he spoke to me as if I did not know anything about operative complications, and tried to shift the blame to the neuroradiologist. He started explaining to me how the brain works and how the coiling procedure had caused this diffuse encephalopathy. Neurologists are frequently called to consult on patients who fail to wake up following surgery. It is an integral part of our specialty to assess brain dysfunction and determine the cause, and, having seen hundreds, if not thousands, of similar cases during my career, I found this patronizing attitude of the anesthesiologist insulting and arrogant.

When I examined Mr. Williams and did another EEG, there was generalized slowing of the brain waves throughout the brain. From these results and his neurological exam findings, it became clear that he had suffered diffuse brain damage from the low blood pressure, which had decreased the blood flow to his brain. This condition is called hypoxic-ischemic encephalopathy or anoxic encephalopathy. This is a very serious problem, and one that is likely to be permanent, with only a small chance of even partial recovery. When general anesthesia is given for any surgical procedure, our body's normal reflexes, which make us breathe and maintain our temperature, blood pressure, and heartbeat are affected, which is why vigilance by the anesthesiologist is so important to maintain blood flow and oxygen to all of our tissues, especially our brains. It is the anesthesiologist's duty to keep us alive during our most vulnerable time in the operating room.

The next step I needed to take was to attempt to explain to the patient's family what was going on and why their husband and father had not woken up following this procedure, which was supposed to save him from the risk of aneurysm rupture and sudden death. I asked the family to gather in a conference room at the end of my hospital rounds, when I could take time to explain what had happened to Mr. Williams, and to answer their questions. "The procedure was a success, but his blood pressure was unstable, and this caused brain damage from which he may not recover," I began. I did not mention that errors had occurred that likely caused the complications he suffered. I did explain that sometimes the brain damage is less severe, and brain cells that are shocked or injured but not dead can resume function, and patients do sometimes wake up within the first few days. I explained that we needed to give him some time to see how much he would recover. I knew that if he did not improve significantly in the first two to three days, his prognosis was dismal, and that he might end up in a persistent vegetative state.

The neuroradiologist on the case came and spoke to the family, but there was a surprising and disappointing lack of communication from the anesthesiologists on the case. As the attending physician, I covered for them as best I could. I was careful to document only the facts, and not my opinion of the situation, in the patient's hospital record. Although I listed "complications of anesthesia" as the cause, I did not list the specifics of how or why that had come about. It was the truth, but I did not ascribe blame to any particular physician or describe the complication as a medical error. Every day I checked on Mr. Williams and sat with Mrs. Williams, holding her hand as I explained that there was little change and that he was unable to come off the breathing machines. After a week, Mr. Williams was still poorly responsive, although there was some brain activity, and he did move spontaneously and withdraw from pain somewhat. This was a slight improvement, although much less than I had hoped for.

We decided that in order to give him more time, a tracheostomy or breathing tube needed to be placed in his neck which could be left in place for a longer time period than the one in his mouth. Because I knew he could not tolerate having this done under general anesthesia and risking another drop in blood pressure, I ordered it to be done under local anesthesia. I spoke to the ENT doctor who would do the procedure. However, on the day of the procedure, the anesthesiologist who was assigned to the case decided to go ahead with the general anesthesia anyway, despite my explicit orders not to. Once again, the patient suffered prolonged low blood pressure, and although the tracheostomy was placed successfully, the patient was delivered back to the ICU in even worse condition, with no responsiveness at all. I could not believe that my direct orders were ignored, and complete disregard for my expertise and judgment was apparent. When I called the anesthesiologist, he was defensive and unwilling to acknowledge any wrongdoing, stating he knew his business better than I, and it was his choice to do whatever he felt best for the patient. When I repeated the EEG, my worst fears were confirmed. What little brain-wave activity had been present before was now flattened out, and the patient was nearly brain dead. He had some primitive brainstem reflexes that allowed his heart to continue beating and exhibited some weak breathing efforts, but the thinking parts of his brain that make us who we are had been destroyed.

Again I called the family together for a conference and plainly told them that the small hope we had clung to for any meaningful recovery was now gone. Worse than that, Mr. Williams could remain in this condition, stuck on life support and comatose for months or even years, in what is called a persistent vegetative state. The family clearly did not want to see their husband and father, who had recently been golfing and enjoying life, in this vegetative state, and the difficult decision of how to allow the end of his life to happen without literally killing him was one that we needed to decide together. As I held Mrs. Williams's hand, we both cried, and I told her how sorry I was that what should have been a life-saving, preventative procedure had gone so terribly wrong. Again, the anesthesiologist who had put the patient under general anesthesia for the tracheostomy never spoke to the family. It was up to me to explain things honestly, but without laying blame on the anesthesiologists involved, in order to avoid a lawsuit, which could easily have come about. Too often, we find ourselves in the uncomfortable position of having to cover for the mistakes made by our colleagues when we talk to patents and their families when a bad outcome occurs, because we have been conditioned to believe that any admission of guilt or error is likely to result in a lawsuit. It is also a fairly common attitude among surgeons and anesthesiologists that they must always be infallible and that they should never acknowledge a mistake. Perhaps they need to convince themselves of their own perfection in order to maintain a steady, confident hand each time they take a patient into surgery. Perhaps their egos are simply unable to tolerate the idea that they, like all human beings, are capable of mistakes that can harm their patients. Perhaps it is the fear of a successful malpractice claim that could end their careers or, at the least, raise their insurance rates to unaffordable levels. In addition, when a physician has a malpractice claim, it follows them for the rest of their lives and is reported to a national practice data bank and must be explained every time the doctor applies for hospital staff privileges, sometimes making it impossible even to qualify for malpractice insurance hospital privileges at all.

What happened next is hard for me to believe, even now. It was an Easter Sunday, and I arrived at the hospital early, hoping to make my rounds on all the hospitalized patients I was covering, and still salvage some of the day for my family. I made my way to the Intensive Care Unit and saw Mr. Williams lying in the bed, oblivious to his surroundings, and still stuck on the ventilator. I saw my other patients and was writing a progress note when a physician I did not know came up to the nursing station and said, "You bitch, I am going to get you fired and kicked off the hospital staff. You will never work anywhere again! You have been telling lies about me, and I am going to put a stop to it! Call the hospital administrator, and we are going to settle this right here and now." I was obviously shocked and replied, "Who are you and what are you talking about?" No fellow physician had ever spoken to me that way, even when I was back in med school studying under some of the toughest, meanest surgical professors in the university. He retorted, "I am the anesthesiologist you slandered in your notes about Mr. Williams, and I am going to get you fired." It took me a while to figure out what he was so upset about, but finally I figured out that he was the one who had completely ignored my direct orders to use a local anesthetic and mild sedation only for the tracheostomy that was placed in Mr Williams for long-term breathing assistance. I was the one who should have been outraged and calling for his termination, after he ignored my direct orders regarding my patient. I had known that the patient would not tolerate another round of general anesthesia, with his brain already in a compromised state, and I had specifically contacted the surgeon who was going to be placing the tracheostomy and spelled out my concerns, and he had agreed to do the procedure that way. I had documented in the chart the orders for local anesthetic only, and had written a progress note explaining the reason for my decision. However, when the time came for the surgery, this anesthesiologist—Dr. Ahole, we'll call him—told the surgeon, "I know what's best for the patient, she doesn't know what she's talking about," and when the surgeon suggested calling me before proceeding, he said, "I don't have time to waste on that. I decide what's best for my patients." The ENT surgeon had told me about his conversation with him.

So, after I was thoroughly cursed out and degraded in the middle of the Intensive Care Unit in front of the nursing staff, the patients, and their families, a hospital administrator was called in for an emergency meeting, and in addition to all my other responsibilities, I was made to sit down with this angry, arrogant individual and discuss the issues regarding my documentation of the plan to try to save Mr. Williams from any further insult to his already traumatized brain—trauma that had been caused by the anesthesia department in the first place. What angered this doctor so much was that I had documented in the patient's chart beforehand that the patient should *not* be placed under general anesthesia for the tracheostomy, and he had done it anyway, making him look bad. He was angry that I might have put him at risk for a malpractice lawsuit. After a two-hour meeting on Easter Sunday, it was decided that a second meeting would be necessary with both the anesthesiology and neurology department heads the next day. Obviously, I was not fired or reprimanded, but it was hard to keep my emotions in check as I continued to see patients and their families the rest of that lovely Easter Sunday, from which I never made it home until late that evening.

The following day, I was called to attend the second meeting with the hospital administrators and department heads to discuss further the situation of poor Mr. Williams and his hypoxic-ischemic encephalopathy. I brought with me the tracings of EEG from before and after the tracheostomy, which clearly showed the changes from slow brain waves to the flat lines that were now present. I reviewed the operative notes from the original procedure, which showed the prolonged periods of hypotension and hypothermia, and the second operative note again showing prolonged periods of hypotension that had knocked off the remaining brain cells the patient had. I stood up for myself and my concern for my patient, while at the same time, I showed that I had not laid blame on the anesthesiologists in the medical record or discussed with the family that medical errors had been made. This relieved the doctors and the hospital administrators more than anything else I said, and after that they were finally satisfied. There was, however, no reprimand for the anesthesiologist or any acknowledgement of fault or error in the management of the case—even behind closed doors. Instead of the case being used to learn from and to prevent further errors like this one, it was swept under the rug. The blame was laid by the anesthesiologists on the neuroradiologist and the aneurysm coiling procedure, even though repeated CT scans showed no stroke or bleed and no obvious complication from the aneurysm. What disappointed me most was the fact that the patient himself was being placed in the background of this risk/liability "crisis." Any honest admission of error and discussion of how it could be avoided in the future was nonexistent. Most important, our role as physicians was fading and had morphed into the personae of businessmen. We had been reduced to bean counters and legal strategists, while our patients and their families suffered in that moment. As I walked away from that second meeting, I rushed to find a place where I could cry unnoticed in a corner of the hospital.

It was shortly after that that I made up my mind to quit working for the multispecialty group. In addition to the above incident, they had neglected to tell me that they were over $30 million in debt and expected me to sign a contract to pay this money back to the local bank. I was not even a partner yet in this group, which had made some very bad corporate decisions, and now they expected me to sign for a debt that most likely would never be paid off in my lifetime. I had never claimed to be much of a businesswoman, but I had a pretty strong feeling that it was time to get out of this relationship with these people who had deceived me and then denigrated me. I turned in my resignation with ninety days' notice just nine months after I had picked up and moved my family, two horses, a dog, and a cat. Because of a strongly worded noncompete clause in my contract, it was clear that if I didn't work for this multispecialty group, I could not stay in town and continue to practice neurology. Their lawyers would have eaten me alive. I even looked into filing a lawsuit against them but the local lawyer I paid several thousand dollars to negotiate with them was of no help. The group terminated my contract on the following Friday by leaving a letter on my desk while I was seeing patients. So I walked out of the building feeling incredulous that my life could have been so thoroughly turned upside down in such a short time and wondering where I would end up next. That very evening, I got a call from the medical director, telling me that they didn't actually think I would leave immediately, even though the letter made it perfectly clear that I was terminated immediately.

He then proceeded to tell me that I was on call that weekend and was expected to cover the hospital and the group's patients for the weekend. He threatened me with the specter of a negative report from the hospital that would stain my career forever, so I had no choice but to go back and take the weekend call. Obviously they had no intention of paying me for this work, and in the end they didn't pay me for that weekend or the entire last month that I had worked. Just to make matters worse, it was the busiest weekend I had ever had on call, and I did twenty-two new neurology consults and followed up on many more of the group's patients who were already in the hospital. I got maybe six hours of sleep the whole weekend long. By the time Monday came, I turned in my reports to the other neurologists and was never so glad to get out of a place as I was then. At that moment I didn't even care that I had no income and no job lined up. Of course it wasn't long before I got more letters asking me to repay this multispecialty group and the hospital over $12,000 for their malpractice tail coverage, my entire previous year's salary, and my moving expenses, for which they had paid. Eventually they sued me, which led to the necessity of filing bankruptcy.

I began a series of interviews, trying to find a job that would be both rewarding and ethical, as well as another place where my family would be happy. We really had liked the area and had made new friends already, but now we had to pack up and move again. As our savings dwindled, I had gotten a taste of a darker side of the health care industry, and it was bitter. It a rude awakening for me, and certainly challenged the idealism I was trying so hard to maintain.

In summary, malpractice is a complex and difficult issue for physicians to deal with on many levels. As consumers of liability insurance, they are subject to the whims of the insurance industry, which sees physicians as prime targets for rate hikes. As practitioners, they have begun to see every patient as a potential lawsuit and have adjusted their practice habits accordingly, even though they are raising the cost of health care exponentially by ordering more tests or procedures than they know are necessary. This practice of defensive medicine does not increase the quality of medical care and adds to the risk of complications by sending physicians and patients on wild-goose chases to follow insignificant or spurious test results. Certain states with higher incidence of lawsuits and without reforms of malpractice laws are seeing an exodus of physicians and shortages of physicians especially in the obstetrics and neurosurgery fields. A single lawsuit can permanently scar the record of an otherwise capable physician, leading him or her to have difficulty changing jobs or moving when trying to obtain affordable insurance in the future. Those who are considering a career in medicine see the malpractice situation as a major deterrent, which is causing us to lose the best and brightest to other careers.

# CHAPTER 5:
## THE DOCTOR AS PATIENT

### DOCTORS MAKE POOR PATIENTS

Most people have heard the cliché that doctors make the worst patients. Nurses probably run a close second. Why would a medical professional be a bad patient? It seems on the surface to be somewhat counterintuitive. After all, they have more knowledge of their condition than the average patient, they are aware of the need for compliance with treatment, and they can communicate with their physicians better in medical terminology. So why don't doctors make the best patients? We are the worst patients in part because we tend to try to control our medical care and interfere with the doctor's and nurse's work, by making our own recommendations for treatment. However, a recent study showed that physicians often recommend different treatments for patients than they would choose for themselves. When it comes to their own health, doctors are often as irrational as everyone else. Physicians often choose against a life saving treatment if it has fewer side effects or complications. (Ubel, Peter, et al. 2011) We often deny that we have a problem as if that would be an admission of weakness. Illness is supposed to happen to someone else, not to us. No amount of doctoring can prepare you for being a patient. Seemingly small annoyances like waiting two hours to see the doctor, or a lab technician having difficulty obtaining blood, become a big deal.

### A LITTLE KNOWLEDGE CAN BE DANGEROUS

I remember when I was in medical school, and I got pregnant for the first time. I had just begun my medical training, but I quickly learned to look up everything I could find on pregnancy and its possible complications. As I gained weight very rapidly, I read about polyhydramnios, an excess of amniotic fluid that often signals a developmental problem with the fetus. When I had tingling in my leg after sitting, I read about nerve root compression. When I didn't feel the baby kick for a few hours, I read about stillbirth, and boy, don't you know I lost some sleep over that one. Every time I caught a cold, I worried about viral effects on a developing fetus. By the time I went to my prenatal visit, I had read up on every symptom I had and all of the possible complications my baby and I could be suffering from.

I was a basket case, and it took quite a bit of reassurance on the part of my physician to convince me that I was just having a normal pregnancy. I questioned everything my doctor told me and wondered if he knew what he was talking about. After all, I was a medical student, and I had read up on all of these disorders of which I had at least one symptom. I must have been a real pain in the neck. Sometimes I got the feeling my doctor considered me just another hysterical female, which didn't help the anxiety I was experiencing. However, he was right, and my baby and I were just fine. They say a little knowledge can be a dangerous thing. Combine that with an overactive imagination, and look out.

In addition, when physicians are trained, most are young and healthy and have not experienced more than a mild or transient illness. They haven't been exposed to the psychology of serious or chronic illness, unless it was through a family member. It is the "really sick people" they treat on a daily basis throughout their careers. Unfortunately there is little training for dealing with the emotional burden of these conditions. Most of us are not prepared to cope with serious illness in our patients, let alone in ourselves.

There are probably few differences in the way doctors react to serious illness from the normal population. However, we tend to hold ourselves to a higher standard than our patients and often expect to continue working and functioning as physicians despite our personal and physical conditions. When we develop symptoms of illness, we often diagnose and treat ourselves in order to avoid being a patient, waiting in another doctor's office and relying on their expertise. Of course the old adage, "A doctor who takes care of himself has a fool for a patient" has remained true to this day.

# DOCTORS HAVE MORE COMPLICATIONS

It is an unwritten rule that doctors and nurses tend to have more complications than normal patients. Although doctors typically think of themselves as indestructible, when they do get sick, they often have rare and unusual conditions. One day the unusual happened to me. I was testing the strength of my patient's legs. This young man had experienced a traumatic brain injury and had little restraint or control over his movements. As I tested his leg strength, he kicked back with his leg so hard and fast that he caught me off guard and off balance. I felt the characteristic pop of a ruptured disc and developed severe pain in my back. The next day I could barely get out of bed, but I still managed to drive myself to work, since I was the attending physician for the hospital neurology service. I had pain, numbness, and tingling running down both legs and noticed I was walking with a definite limp, as my right ankle was weak. I did my best to ignore the pain and continued to work, knowing that the patients and my colleagues depended on me. Calling in sick was simply not an option. As I made my one-hour commute, the pain in my legs was almost unbearable, but I kept hoping it would go away when I got busy and distracted myself from it. Over the next few days, I got some steroids and tried those to relieve some of the inflammation. I took ibuprofen every few hours. I held out for two weeks, but as the right foot drop worsened, I finally decided to see a colleague who was a neurosurgeon. He ordered an MRI of my back before seeing me the following week. When I went in, I felt awkward sitting in the waiting room, MRI films in hand, filling out the reams of paperwork required. Of course I had reviewed the MRI myself before going in, and I had an idea what was going to happen, but it felt so wrong being in the patient's position this time. As I was led back to an exam room, I sat trying to compose my thoughts, calm my nerves, and condense all the symptoms I had been experiencing into a cohesive history. It seemed like it all went out the window when the doctor came in. I stammered and stuttered through the visit, forgetting half of the symptoms I wanted to tell him about. I realized with some chagrin that this anxiety is how my patients often feel when they come in to see me. As the doctor examined me I worried that my feet smelled or that he thought I was fat. He recommended a trial of physical therapy and epidural steroids, which is what I had figured on, but squeezing all that into my normal twelve-hour workday was going to be tricky. I managed to get the therapy done in the early mornings before patients arrived and the injections during the lunch hour. After an epidural steroid injection, it is difficult to go back to work, attempting to bend and twist as before, but I didn't want to inconvenience the patients who had come a long way and waited for an appointment to see me. In between patients, I banged my head against the wall. I was determined to tough it out. I composed myself and put on my best professional face, trying to concentrate fully on the next patient's symptoms.

After six weeks of conservative therapy, I still had a pronounced foot drop, and I knew this was more serious than a muscular strain of my back. I headed back to the neurosurgeon, and he scheduled me for surgery. The next two weeks of anticipation allowed me time to review all the possible complications of spine surgery, but I reassured myself that they could never happen to me. After all, the chances of complications were very low for a routine laminectomy. Basically, an incision is made in the back and a piece of the vertebral bone is removed. This allows access to the inner spinal column, where the ruptured disc can be removed, and the nerve roots freed up. I planned to return to work in a month and was reassured by my office that I would continue to be paid on short-term disability for that month.

I arrived for surgery with my husband on a Monday morning, having eaten and drank nothing, per instructions. The waiting room had several patients who were having surgery that morning, and we were all herded into the elevators like so many cattle to the preop holding room. The nurses seemed very cold and disinterested; no one smiled or made simple conversation, and my nerves were really on edge by now. Soon they came and put in an IV, and the surgeon made his brief pre-op appearance. He reassured me everything would be fine. They put a sedative in my IV, and the next thing I knew, the surgery was over. The surgeon was talking to me, saying something about a dural tear. He had accidentally made a hole in the membrane surrounding the spinal nerves, which he spent an extra thirty minutes sewing up. I had to lie flat on my back for the next twenty-four hours, however. I was so groggy I didn't really care. I slept through most of that day. The next day they pulled out the catheter in my bladder, and I got up to go to the bathroom. Strangely, I couldn't pee normally, and when I wiped myself I couldn't feel anything on my buttocks or perineum. I thought, *No problem. They must have given me a saddle block for the surgery.* However, when the anesthesiologist came to check on me, he denied having given me any local anesthetic, and when the surgical resident came in, he denied it too. I reported the numbness

I had, and they scheduled another MRI of my spine, which wasn't done until the next day. It was done in the afternoon, and following that, the nurses put a catheter back in my bladder, which showed a large amount of retained urine. Being a neurologist, I knew all too well the implications of this. I had cauda equina syndrome. This meant damage to the nerves that control the bowel, bladder, and sexual function. The neurosurgeon returned and informed me that I had an epidural hematoma, or blood clot, compressing my spinal canal and the nerves in my lower back. He then took a long spinal needle and while I lay there in the bed, he tried to drain the fluid collection he had seen on the MRI. After several pokes with a long spinal needle and considerable pain, he informed me that he had to re-operate on my back. This blood clot had formed just outside the spinal canal and was causing my symptoms. As I tried to prepare myself for a second surgery on Day Two, I cried, wondering, as people often do, "Why me?" This was an extremely rare complication of a simple laminectomy. I was supposed to go home the same day and back to work in a month. I felt like the Queen of Irony.

They came for me that evening, and back to the cold, sterile operating room I went. I vaguely remember waking up and hearing the surgeon say that they got the clot out, but another twenty-four hours flat on my back was required. When you have just had two surgeries on your back, the last position you want to be in is lying on your back. I was miserable, but I tried to tolerate the discomfort in a mature way, kicking and griping whenever the sedatives and morphine wore off. The following day, I was again allowed to get up, and went to the bathroom to try unsuccessfully for a bowel movement, which was now three days overdue. However, this time when I got up, I developed the worst headache I had ever experienced in my life. It was as though an elephant had sat on my head. I felt like my brain was squeezing out through my ears and down my neck. I barely made it back to bed, and as I lay down, the headache eased up. "Wow, this is interesting," I thought. As I lay there and analyzed the situation, I recognized from my patients' description of similar symptoms that this was a spinal headache, a complication I had seen and even caused a few times by doing spinal taps on some patients. Having never experienced anything like this before, I now gained a new sense of appreciation for the meaning of the word *headache*. The back pain paled in comparison. The outside world paled in comparison. As I threw up, I knew that I had a big problem. I remembered with horror the surgeon telling me about the dural tear he had caused during the first surgery. Later that day, the surgeon came in to make his rounds, and I told him about the headache. He was clearly upset but said, "No problem, it's just a small CSF leak, it will clear up in a few days." I couldn't even stand up at all without the rapid onset of this ten out of ten headache, however, and even lying down, it was at least a seven. I lay there in the hospital for another three days, without even being seen by an attending doctor—only a five-minute visit from the resident each day. I thought, "They've given up on me. If they treat me this way, and I am a colleague, how do they treat their other patients?"

When it became clear that the surgeon had no further plans for me, I was discharged via ambulance back home, with home health and my husband to take care of me. I went from industrious to invalid in the course of one week. I went from bed to couch to bathroom, carrying a bag full of urine attached to my catheter. I watched daytime TV in a daze of pain medications. I reveled in finally getting my hair washed, in the bed, by a nurse's aide, after nine days of blood, sweat, and tears. Having to get your butt washed by a stranger, even if she is medical personnel, is a unique patient-related experience, and not one I would care to repeat. The only other time I was in that situation I was too young to know any better.

I had worked sixty to eighty hours a week in a dignified position at the university, and now it began to hit me how sick I really was. I was having horrible headaches, and I couldn't stand more than a few minutes without feeling like passing out. My back was so tender, I couldn't stand to wear clothes. I lived in my nightgowns for two months. To try to get out of bed and walk outside was a full day's effort, and one for which I paid dearly. I couldn't pee and had to take a handful of medications just to get by. I got a urinary tract infection. I was a handful for home health and my husband. Thank God that I have a husband who was willing and able to devote his energy to my needs. However, despite his care I continued to deteriorate, with worsening headaches and weakness. I was taken back to the hospital by ambulance a week after discharge. They scanned my head and my back. The surgeon said, "It's not that bad," and sent me back home. Two days later, my headaches let up a little, but I traded them for a new pain, which ran down my left hip and the back of my leg. When I tried to stand up, it felt like rubber bands snapping in my thigh. Any movement, especially going to the bathroom, was excruciating. My doctor told me he was "too invested" in my case. I thought, *That's the last thing I wanted to hear from the doctor who put me in this condition.* He said he had discussed my case with his colleagues and that there was nothing more he could do. He said that I would probably be disabled for at least six months, but that eventually I *might* get better. He sent me home, having done nothing except give me pain medication. He simply recommended I wait it out, and eventually it should get better. I couldn't bend or stoop at all, so I walked a few minutes at a time with a cane in one hand and a "grabber" in the other. I got a toilet seat extension, which helped me not sit so far back on the seat, and I couldn't sit in a chair at all, even with a wheelchair cushion. My husband brought me all my meals in bed or on the couch. The incontinence was the most embarrassing and humiliating condition, however. I spent 98 percent of my time all summer lying down in the bed or the couch watching TV. The other two percent was spent in the bathroom. "This is it?" I asked myself. "This is what I have to look forward to for the next six months?" I remember telling the husband to go get me a knife and a pillow, so I could stab something without causing too much harm.

The worst feeling was when I returned to my doctor about the headaches and the severe back pain. He seemed to downplay my symptoms and blame them on sacroiliac joint inflammation and rebound headaches. Rebound headaches are usually caused by withdrawal of narcotic medications when people have been taking them for a long time. As a neurologist, I have quite a bit of expertise in headaches. These headaches, associated with standing up, were typical of spinal headaches. The pain from my back radiating into the posterior thigh was typical of nerve root pain. I had pulsatile tinnitus, a ringing in the ears associated with the heart beat, especially when I stood up or rolled over. Yet, I could not get this doctor to see that there was something seriously wrong. I realized again that many patients feel put off by their doctors, who discount their symptoms or simply don't believe them. After phone calls and e-mails to this doctor for several more weeks, I insisted on getting an urgently scheduled appointment. When I arrived, the nurse in the clinic remarked that he was in surgery and might be a few minutes late. She put me in a room where I could lie on an exam table, since I couldn't sit. I waited there for two hours, and he never showed up. The nurse never even came back to check me or to tell me the doctor was still busy. I had a spell of nearly passing out when I rolled over, and finally, I couldn't take it anymore. I told my husband to take me home. The next day, I scheduled a second opinion with a neurologist and a different neurosurgeon. I had known and trusted him from my years of private practice. He had helped many of my patients in the past, and I prayed that he could help me. Nonetheless, I felt my life slipping away, and I realized that I would never be normal again. A strong depression began to seep into my heart, and I prepared myself for death. I had all but given up. I even looked forward to being put out of my misery and pain.

After another week of lying in the bed, being catheterized twice a day by home health, I saw a neurologist, who was also a friend. When I stood up and he saw the way my lower back swelled up, he was shocked. It was obvious to him what was going on; he said I had a pseudomeningocele, and the only remedy would be a third surgery. I began to cry, not only out of fear of more surgery, but from the relief that finally someone believed me, and that there was a legitimate reason for the way I felt. He referred me to the neurosurgeon who had treated many of my patients successfully. The neurosurgeon also said it was obvious that I had a large pseudomeningocele. This is a pocket or cyst filled with spinal fluid that is connected to the spinal column. The neurosurgeon didn't need an MRI to see what was going on. The only way to fix the problem was to re-operate, remove the pseudomeningocele and its capsule, reapproximate the muscles that had been displaced, and find the hole in the dura where the spinal fluid was leaking out and sew it up.

It took another two weeks for the original neurosurgeon and the second neurosurgeon to contact each other and for the first one to release me to be treated by the other. The first surgeon's office staff kept telling the second surgeon's office that he was out of town. I don't know the reason he was avoiding the call, but I was in the middle of a mess, and I just wanted to get on with treatment. After several more phone calls back and forth, I finally got a date for the third surgery. I continued to feel myself deteriorating on a daily basis and could not do anything for myself. I was having more of the spells where I would nearly pass out when changing positions. Finally the date came, two months after the second surgery, for repair of the spinal fluid–filled pseudomeningocele. The third surgery went pretty well, and the neurosurgeon told me that I had a gallon of spinal fluid in my back. When he made the first incision in my skin, he said my spinal fluid made a foot-high fountain as it drained. Not only did he find a huge hole in my dura, he also found that my nerve roots were entrapped and kinked like an elbow in the opening. This explained a lot of the rubber band-like nerve pain I was experiencing in my leg. He was able to repair all that successfully, however, and felt very positive about my outcome. Over the next week, I still had the most awful headaches and still had the pain in my leg and back. Gradually, over the next couple of weeks, the pain seemed to ease up some, however, and I was able to walk a little with the cane. However, when I tried to do physical therapy, the pain all came back, including the headaches. I had a recurrence of pulsatile tinnitus. Every time I sat for any length of time and stood up again, my hearing would go in and out like a wah-wah pedal, which correlated to my heart beat. I would get dizzy and have to wait until it passed, which usually took a minute or so. I continued to have the bowel and bladder problems and had lost my sexual function as well. Although this was clearly an uncomfortable topic for my doctors, it was a major quality-of-life issue for me. Although we study sexuality in medical school, we are still as a whole uncomfortable talking about it to our patients. From a patient's standpoint, our doctors are often the only person with whom we might feel comfortable talking about sexuality if we are asked about it. Unfortunately, despite multiple treatments available for male sexual dysfunction, there is nothing available that is effective for females.

Over the next several months, my symptoms persisted, although the pain gradually diminished, and I was able to get off the daily pain-killers. I had a strong fear of becoming addicted to narcotics, and yet, in my condition, I could see how so many patients got that way. Chronic daily pain that you can't escape is a condition that no one should have to experience, yet there are hundreds of thousands of people in similar situations across the country who are addicted to Oxycontin, morphine, or hydrocodone. The problem with these drugs is that they become less effective as they are taken daily—a phenomenon called tolerance. The pain actually intensifies, and of course nothing relieves it but stronger and more frequent doses of the narcotics. I was determined not to get into the narcotic rat race and get labeled by my fellow physicians as a "drug-seeker." I held myself to that higher standard that physicians are supposed to maintain. I tried to suffer with the pain rather than take the pills.

I was also getting hooked on sleeping pills, since the pain would wake me up every night, and I could not get comfortable. In addition, I would spend nights worrying about what was going to happen to me and whether I would ever be up well enough to work again. I wondered how I was going to support my family and whether or not we would ever recover financially from this. I had always been the sole supporter for my family, the strong one, the one on whom everyone else relied. When I had left work for this first surgery, I was told that I would continue to be paid under short-term disability benefits. However, a month into my illness, my employer sent me a letter saying that my salary would be cut because I was not able to produce. This cut my paycheck down to one-third of normal. Fortunately, I had had the sense to keep a personal disability policy in place since my residency. This is a very important insurance policy anyone with a substantial income should have, especially with occupation-specific coverage.

Finally, my employment at the university was terminated. My doctor told me it would probably be at least a year before I'd be able to return to work, and even that was questionable. All those months with spinal fluid leak, three surgeries, and inflammation had also taken their toll on my memory. At first I could barely put two words together to make a sentence, but eventually I started to be able to speak fairly normally. However I was having trouble doing simple activities around the house that normally came easily. I could not hold on to a single thought. I had trouble remembering the names and dosages of my own medications. How could I treat patients when I couldn't remember even simple things like conversations? It seemed like all the years of studying and practicing medicine had all gone out the window. I had a justifiable fear of hurting or killing someone by making a simple or obvious mistake because of my condition.

I continued to have problems as the days slowly passed. Although the pain was a little better, I still had dizzy spells every time I stood up and headaches that would just become unbearable by the end of the day. Finally I could relate to my patients who complained of headaches that would lay them out. I developed greater compassion for my patients who were disabled. I knew the frustration of wanting to work and being unable to do so. In an instant I had lost my health, my career and most of the hobbies that I had loved to do. I questioned my purpose in life in a way that I had never done before. How could I help anyone anymore when I couldn't even help myself?

They say things happen for a reason. There are many physicians who are going out on disability or quitting altogether and closing their doors. I have certainly experienced the frustrations trying to practice good medicine in a bad system. However, the joy of helping others always outweighed the bad. Now that I was physically unable to carry out my job, I missed my sense of purpose and the challenge from each day with my patients. I missed my patients and the relationships I had with them as well as with my office staff and other physicians. Now that I had been transformed into a chronic pain patient, I decided that I liked it better on the other end of the stethoscope.

Before I got sick, I had started working on this book. During the worst of my illness, I was unable to work on it because I was unable to sit at the computer or to think clearly. I tried to study my neurology journals, but everything I read seemed to go in one ear and out the other. My worst fears of being incompetent seemed to be coming true. If I went back to practicing medicine, would I kill someone or harm them by forgetting a side effect or a drug interaction or by giving the wrong dosage? Or would I reinjure my back and have to cancel all the patient appointments I had and go back on disability within a few months of resuming practice? I had to learn to take one day at a time, and gradually I got better. After much soul searching, I came to accept that although I could no longer practice clinical neurology, I could write, I could stand up and fight for the causes I never had time for before, I could spend more time with my family, and I could find a new purpose for my life.

## BEING A PATIENT MAKES A BETTER DOCTOR

On the day that my mother died after a prolonged hospital stay, I made rounds on my hospital patients and tried to devote all my attention to those in my care. I couldn't allow myself the luxury of experiencing the grief that welled up inside me or to ask for help. My patients and their families had enough to deal with without knowing about my problems, and they needed me. I summoned up every bit of strength I had to concentrate on my patients' exams, labs, imaging studies, and vital signs. I hope I did the right thing, but at what cost? Where was my family, where were my kids, during those difficult times while I was away at the hospital?

As good physicians, we try to empathize with our patients, but it is very difficult fully to understand disease and its impact on our patients until it happens to us. It can be a severe emotional drain to get too close to our patients' problems and still function objectively as their physician. We have to shield our emotions from the reality of disease, pain, and death that we see on a daily basis in order to keep from being swept up in the whirlwind and lose our focus on practicing good medicine. We must be somewhat hardened to the pain and suffering around us in order to have the strength to carry on in our professions. Yet, when physicians get seriously ill, we cannot separate our emotions from our physical bodies. We often cannot accept that we may have to stop and experience the pain of a serious illness that may limit our activities. We must lower our expectations of ourselves as the strong ones, always caring for others rather than ourselves. We are confronted with the fact that we are imperfect; that we cannot be and do everything, despite years of programming that we must. In the setting of a serious illness, this realization can come to a crisis that affects the way a doctor behaves as a patient. We may deny warning signs of illness or refuse to take medications that would force us to acknowledge the problem. We may self-medicate to avoid making a trip to a doctor. We may get frustrated and take our anger out on family, friends, and our patients. We often get depressed, feeling betrayed by our bodies, and may lose hope of returning to our normally busy, intense lives.

When we become disabled, we find that we are not qualified to do anything else but practice our specialty. This really limits us when we are forced to consider alternatives to our regular jobs. We have to be able to give one 110 percent to our medical jobs every day, or we risk making a mistake that could harm a patient. When we become patients, we can no longer give of ourselves to this extent.

If we do recover and return to the practice of medicine, however, it is with a renewed sense of empathy for our patients, and that makes us better physicians. We see our role in caring for patients differently. We spend more time explaining the disease and the patient's options with a greater focus on the patient's quality of life than the statistical probability that they will respond to a given treatment. We make recommendations and explain the risks and benefits, but recognize that the final decision must be up to the patient. Our understanding of pain, illness and death is broadened and our role in helping to alleviate suffering clarified. **If anything, it's that recognition of vulnerability in illness, as well as their expertise that makes physicians better doctors.** Despite the pain and suffering I experienced, having these medical problems has been an enlightening journey to the patient's end of the stethoscope.

# CHAPTER 6:
## THE FUTURE OF MEDICINE—
## A PHYSICIAN'S PERSPECTIVE

As we embrace the second millennium, physicians look at the future of medicine in America, as well as to our careers and our personal lives. If things continue as they are now, ominous signs portend more difficult times for both physicians and their patients. Surely, there are some good things on the horizon, with the possibility of new treatments for diseases we cannot cure now and legislation to cover more Americans with health insurance. However, the costs of medical care and innovative treatments in the future may bankrupt the country and its citizens if something is not done. What good will life-saving treatments be if no one can afford them? Rising costs and decreasing reimbursement threaten to bankrupt physicians and make a career in medicine less and less desirable. What good will all the high-tech innovations, expanded health care insurance and new medications be if there are not enough doctors to administer them? Widespread shortages of physicians will be exacerbated by the coverage of all citizens, making waiting times more lengthy, and straining the physician-patient relationship further. As young people head out to college, they will weigh the pros and cons of a medical education, and many promising doctors will opt out for other careers, unless something is done to improve the benefits and reduce the risk sides of the equation. This is a time when we should be encouraging more young people to choose a career in medicine to accommodate our baby-boomer generation's increased health care needs. Instead, our current system is making it harder and harder for physicians and those who are considering a career in medicine. As I mentioned earlier, studies show that most physicians no longer recommend their careers to their families or friends, and many are leaving the medical field at unprecedented rates.

How can we as a society and as individuals support our nation's physicians, making their jobs more about medical care, respect, and appreciation, and less about paperwork, regulations, and legal liabilities?

The Obama Health Care Plan, or the Patient Protection and Affordable Care Act (PPACA), a historic piece of legislation, was approved on March 23, 2010, with provisions that are to be phased in through 2014 (Patient Protection and Affordable Care Act HR03590, 2010). The main thrust of this plan is to require and support health insurance for all Americans. The plan also includes some much needed regulations on the private health insurance companies. These include better coverage in 2014 for those with preexisting conditions without gouging patients on the rates. There will be subsidies for low-income families who cannot afford a premium, but with an expected rise in healthy populations that formerly did without insurance, the profits of insurance companies are still likely to be secure. In actuality, rates should go down for everyone because of an improved risk pool requiring fewer overall costs. It was unlikely, however, that the insurance companies would voluntarily refund or reduce anyone's insurance premium, so part of the bill also includes a mandate that administrative costs are to be limited to twenty percent instead of the thirty-one percent insurance companies now claim to pay for the CEOs exorbitant salaries and fancy offices.

Having worked in the managed care field, I saw firsthand how much radiology managed care could save an insurance company, and I felt like I was doing some good in cutting down health care costs. Unfortunately, those savings were not passed on to the consumer, and health insurance rates were increased across the board and across various insurance companies. Stockholders were happy with the record profits these companies have had, but the time has come for insurance companies to stop breaking the backs of physicians and their patients to line their pockets. Corporate greed in health care is killing our patients and our profession. The federal government may not be perfect, but at least it is not in health care to make a profit. Medicare and Medicaid have been pretty effective and beneficial programs for all these years, although their existence is threatened by the recent economic downturn and the aging baby-boomer population. Ask anyone who has his or her health care through one of these programs, and you will see that they are a lifeline for many people in this country, who otherwise would be literally dying in the streets. While it is not clear what all the ramifications of the new health care plan will be, it will be a benefit to physicians to be paid for more of the patients they see, even the two AM ER consult that previously went unpaid. Since most people will have some form of health insurance coverage, they will be more likely to go to the outpatient clinic during business hours, and before their condition has gotten out of control.

With the passage of the health reform act in 2010, many new regulations and requirements are being phased in that will affect all physicians, but especially those in private practice. In a survey by Merritt Hawkins, most physicians responded unfavorably to the passage of the health reform bill, because they see it further increasing their patient loads while decreasing reimbursement. They see a drastic increase in legal compliance obligations, increased oversight and decreased reimbursement, a formula that will likely drive the remaining independent private practice physicians out of business, or into some type of employment with a large group, hospital, or Accountable Care Organization (ACO) (The Physicians Foundation, 2008). In another survey of physicians in response to the Affordable Care Act, the majority of physicians (60%) said health reform will compel them to close or restrict their practices to certain categories of patients. Of these, 93% said they will close or significantly restrict their practices to Medicaid patients, while 87% said they would close or significantly restrict their practices to Medicare patients. In response to reform, 40% of physicians said they would drop out of patient care in the next one to three years, either by retiring, seeking a non-clinical job within healthcare, or by seeking a non-healthcare related job. (The Physicians Foundation, 2010) If the government could just simplify the paperwork rather than increasing it, and back off on the micromanagement, physicians might just have a chance at returning to what they love—practicing medicine.

## PRESERVING HUMANITY IN MEDICINE

The individual patient and his or her doctor are getting lost in the whirlwind of changes in computerization, mechanization, regulation, and technology. The art and the joy of medicine and the doctor-patient relationship are disappearing as our patients find themselves standing before a computer that pokes and prods them, scans them, spits out a diagnosis and a prescription and then sends them on their way. Internet physicians are writing prescriptions for potentially dangerous medicines as patients attempt to treat themselves, rather than going to their physicians for a proper diagnosis and selective treatment. People are buying so-called "life scans," subjecting themselves to radiation and unnecessary costs in order to self-diagnose, when they really don't need these tests. Is this really what we want from our health care system? Will medical mistakes be any less common in a system like this?

Many of the "old school" docs will struggle not to get lost in the whirlwind of changes coming about. It seems already that the good, old-fashioned history and examination are a thing of the past. Instead of taking time to talk to the patients, explain a diagnosis and its implications, we rush through the patient encounter to keep up with our hectic schedules. Instead of answering questions, we may hand out a paper on the patients' condition, which may or may not be understandable or helpful in answering the patient's questions. We do our fancy, computer-driven histories and physicals with fill-in-the-blanks formats. This certainly doesn't provide the empathy or compassion people expect and need from their physicians. The benefits of technology, such as electronic medical records and electronic prescriptions, have been tremendous assets in reducing medical errors; however, we need to remember to look our patient in the eyes and establish a line of communication and trust where the true healing occurs. We must know our patients by name, not by diagnosis.

## ART VS. SCIENCE IN MEDICINE

Scientific study is expanding our overall knowledge in so many areas of medicine simultaneously that it is impossible for any physician to keep up with it all, even in their chosen specialty, especially when we are working sixty to one hundred hours per week treating patients. Physicians do the best they can, attending medical conferences throughout the year that review the most clinically relevant breakthroughs or advances. They continue to read up on the subjects presented by their patients with their various clinical symptoms. When they arrive at a diagnosis, they try to stay abreast of the latest or best treatments for that disease. However, in their hearts they know that there is always someone who knows more about a given subject, someone who is smarter, faster, and more proficient than they are. There is always a sense of chasing after a speeding train, always trying to catch up to the most current state of knowledge and skill. There is also a part of them that realizes that, even with the best available knowledge, there is so much yet unknown about medicine and all the individual factors that go into treating their patients, scientific perfection in medicine can never be achieved.

There is more art than science in most fields of medicine today. The simple act of touching our patients when we greet them, examine them, and leave them cannot be underestimated in its therapeutic value. If it is true that nearly one-third of patients enrolled in a double-blinded clinical research study will respond to the treatment given, even though it is a placebo, how do we physicians harness this tremendous benefit and take advantage of the incredible healing potential of the mind? As I have mentioned, I spent a year or two practicing a form of massage prior to entering medical school and saw firsthand the powerful effects of human touch. As a neurologist, I have seen the healing that comes from simply being a good listener and providing empathy to my patients who were stuck in life's struggles with bottled-up frustrations and worries. Many times it was just the recognition that stress was causing their unusual symptoms that allowed those symptoms to dissipate, and to have a physician touch them and let them know they were not alone made all the difference. No computer diagnostic program, powerful as it may be, will be successful at replacing the healing art of health care. Yet when the reimbursement system rewards the volume of patients seen rather than being a caring, compassionate physician who takes the time to listen to and examine their patients, explaining the medical condition and treatment options, the quality of America's health care will continue to go down, and patients will feel more and more like herds of cattle, while physicians feel more like administrators of health care than healers.

## THE DOCTOR-PATIENT RELATIONSHIP— ADVERSARIES OR ALLIES?

In the final analysis, physicians are fighting against the nature of human beings, which is to be born and to die. When it is one's time to die, no physician can stand in the way of fate, although we try to do so every day. Like the proverbial knight on a big white horse, we see ourselves standing up to the thirty-foot dragon of disease. Sometimes we win the battle, and at other times the dragon wins. In the end, despite our best efforts, death eventually wins every time. The best physicians can hope for is to delay the inevitable. While this may seem to be a dramatized depiction of our jobs, I believe that most physicians do feel something like knights in shining armor. There have also been many times I felt as if I was standing in front of a speeding train with some of my sicker patients.

When we choose a medical career, we go off to work each day to fight trauma, disease, and death. It is much more than a job; it is a destiny, a true calling. Some people accuse physicians of thinking they are God. I like to think of it more as though we are using our God-given talents to reverse the natural course of events that through illness or injury would otherwise occur. Many times we simply feel like witnesses to the hand of God as it touches our patients. I have seen many inexplicable cases where against all odds the patient lived. I have also seen those times where, although the patient looked well on paper, he or she died with no medical explanation. I have seen patients rise up like Lazarus after being declared dead. In reality, physicians have very little control and very little knowledge in the big picture of life and death.

We can often improve the quality of life through our treatments, even for incurable diseases, and our treatments can prolong life for years. We continue to probe the unknown through scientific research, making strides every year in finding causes and treatments for illnesses that have plagued humankind since time began, as well as for new diseases that have developed more recently, such as swine flu or AIDS.

Perhaps I should have picked an easier career than medicine. I felt the calling to this challenging career, and a need to do something of service to mankind. However, it got more and more difficult to get up on that horse each day and ride off toward the battles that lay ahead. The difficulties of practicing medicine—with the paperwork, the overhead costs, dealing with insurance companies, and the liability issues—began to out-shadow the joy of helping and healing others. When we have to see patients every five or ten minutes to keep our doors open, it is easy to lose sight of the reasons we went into medicine. If patients feel like herds of cattle, imagine how the cattle herder feels. "Next!" we cry, as our staff hurry people in one exam room and out another. Many physicians out there are also feeling this frustration and are retiring early. Because I am a physician, I am not qualified to do much else but medicine. Many physicians feel trapped in their careers and would choose another career if given a choice or another lifetime.

In fact, when I initially became disabled but got well enough to walk and function somewhat, I tried to get a job teaching nurses at two local colleges and was soundly rejected because I don't have a nursing degree. My MD degree didn't qualify me for any other medical career. Even being a neurologist didn't qualify me to work in any other field of medicine, like primary care. When we do such a specialized thing, we are put in a niche that we often have trouble wiggling out of. There has been much talk of making it easier for professionals to go back to the classroom to share their knowledge and experience with students, but this has not really come about to any great extent, at least in my experience. I finally found work in radiology managed care, reviewing medical information and making a determination of the appropriateness of requested imaging studies. It opened my eyes to a subculture of medical professionals who have turned to imaging tests like CT and MRI as an alternative to performing a detailed history and physical examination. It showed me how severe the consequences of practicing defensive medicine can be and why the health care costs have gone up so much. Many physicians have found that ownership of imaging equipment can be a lucrative business, supplementing the decreasing reimbursement that routine office care provides. However, as payments for this expensive equipment must be made, the likelihood that a physician who owns this equipment will order excessive testing increases.

In addition, talking with physicians across the country while doing this work has shown me that physicians out there are fearful of missing a rare disease, however unlikely, and losing their livelihood in a lawsuit. This fear outweighs common sense and good judgment when it comes to ordering tests or helping to control the cost of medical care. Until physicians feel safe to practice medicine as they were taught, to consider how or whether a test will be likely to change the management of a patient, defensive medicine, a major cause of rising health care costs, will continue to worsen. Micromanagement of physicians is not the answer.

Part of our role as physicians is to accept responsibilities and our own limitations in this battle for our patients' health. Although we are not perfect, we jump in and do the best we can. We make our diagnoses based on statistics from prior research, while distilling the history, examination, and testing results to reveal the most likely condition. We treat with medications that are shown to be effective in a majority of patients and hope that a given patient will not be in the small percentage who has serious side effects or no benefit at all. The American public must realize and accept that no human can take on all the duties we physicians try to tackle each day without some errors. We make errors of omission and commission on a regular basis, although the vast majority of these errors are minor and don't affect our patient's health. If we were sued for all the mistakes we make, all physicians would be out of business within a year.

Many errors can be corrected without long-term complications when brought to our attention. When physicians and their patients keep the lines of communication open, they are able to react more quickly and respond to the changes that occur in a disease process. We can correct errors before they get out of hand. The greatest tool in the reduction of medical errors has been the establishment of a system of checks and balances, where multiple people are looking at a given prescription, for example, and verifying its accuracy and appropriateness. Now when a patient goes to surgery, the physician will mark the area to be operated on while the patient looks on and agrees. The nurses on the floor and in the operating room will verify with the patient the planned procedure and review the hospital chart. Before the anesthesiologist puts the patient to sleep, he or she will also verify the correctness of the planned procedure and any allergies to medications. It is this repetition of checks by multiple individuals that helps to ensure that a mistake is caught before a grave complication can occur. Similarly, documentation with electronic medical records is helping to eliminate errors by providing a way for clear, typewritten notes to be made available to other physicians caring for a patient, to insurance companies, and to hospitals or other medical facilities involved in a patient's care. Electronic prescriptions that are double-checked by pharmacists help to eliminate the error of incorrect medications or dosages being prescribed to patients. These programs are saving health care dollars by reducing errors and duplicate testing or prescriptions. By improving access to medical records, treating physicians can be aware of prior workups for a given problem, see what has been done for the patient by other physicians, and avoid drug interactions or allergic reactions and unnecessary treatments.

While managed care is most likely a necessary evil in today's world, it could be handled in better ways. Instead of physician panels of reviewers on insurance company or managed care company payrolls that review and decide on requests from all areas of medicine, a single-payer system would allow for a larger, single board of physicians who review cases for appropriateness and quality of care, within their individual specialties. This would not only insure a higher level of quality in the managed care process, it would provide a venue through the specialty society's educational programs to retrain physicians and correct the problem at its source. By creating clear-cut standards of care and practice management guidelines, poor outcomes that occur despite a physician's best treatment within these standards would not be subject to as great a risk of a successful malpractice lawsuit. The specialty societies could also direct the outlying physician to specific coursework related to the errors or omissions identified in a physician's performance. Oversight of physician activities is a necessary part of the process as well, to identify and correct those doctors with practices that fall outside the standards of care as defined by specialty societies, medical training, or medical ethics. However, it is not lawyers or dissatisfied patients who are going to correct a problem with an outlying physician. Punitive damages are not the answer for retraining physicians.

At the same time, we cannot continue to make the practice of medicine so cumbersome and time-consuming that it is no longer efficient or tolerable for physicians. We must make this career an attractive vocation again, and one in which we are still recruiting the best and the brightest minds to devote themselves to healing, solving the medical problems of the day, and serving others in such a noble way. If we take the joy of medicine away, who will be willing to make the sacrifices involved in being a physician?

The future of medicine in America seems pretty frightening to me these days. Everywhere I look, I see major problems with a system that needs radical change. While the Affordable Care Act has some provisions that will benefit patients and protect them from some of the price gouging insurance and pharmaceutical companies, most physicians see it as adding more layers of complexity, reducing the quality of health care, and not solving the underlying problems of a for-profit health care system. Yet, there are powerful political forces out there that are working to maintain the status quo. The only status quo I believe physicians want is to preserve the dignity and closeness of the doctor-patient relationship, and to earn what allows us to live a comfortable lifestyle. No physician would choose this career simply for the money. We are humanitarians first; good will and brotherly love drive us to participate in the health care of others. Respect, honor and appreciation from our patients are the best rewards we can achieve. The intellectual challenges of medicine are enough to fulfill even the most brilliant minds. Of course we expect to be paid for our work, and to make a decent living, after all the education, hard work and sacrifice of our personal lives to care for the sick. Unfortunately, more and more patients come to us with an attitude of doubt and suspicion, and an expectation that we should provide quick and easy cures with perfection in all cases. When confronted with these attitudes, it is harder to give all of yourself into a relationship. It is hard not to become cynical and mistrustful in these times. The incredible idealism with which we started our careers is too often left by the wayside as we confront the realities of practicing medicine in the twenty-first century.

So, what can we do about the current health care crisis? What kinds of solutions are available to us in order to improve health care in America? How can we pull ourselves out of this crisis and improve the quality of health care for all Americans, not just for the privileged few? There are lots of great ideas out there, and other countries have set examples of national health care systems that we could borrow from in creating a system that is best for America. What kind of solution is available to us to improve health care for all Americans? How can we provide quality health care without going bankrupt as a nation or as individual patients and physicians?

## GETTING CONTROL OVER THE MIDDLEMEN

The costs of health care are often blamed on physicians. However, as discussed earlier, the majority of our health care dollars are spent on pharmaceutical and medical supply companies, insurance companies, and lawyers. Physicians are caught in the middle and are feeling the squeeze on both the income and expense sides of the equation. We want our patients to have the benefits of the latest discoveries and treatments for their medical conditions. However, these new treatments continue to drive up the costs of health care. Physicians have no control over what pharmaceutical and medical supply companies charge and receive no kickbacks for ordering a newer, more expensive treatment. Why not consider restricting the profit margins of these companies or placing caps on the prices we are willing to pay for new medicines or treatments? Why not enforce the patent expiration dates on brand-name medications without exceptions, so less expensive generics are more readily available? Why not insist that Americans pay the same cost for the same medications as other countries? The government is willing to step into private enterprise when it involves a national, indispensable need. They have done so in the transportation industry, communications, food, environmental protection, and in many other areas. Physician's activities have been regulated to an extreme degree already, from both a quality as well as a reimbursement standpoint. Regulation of hospitals' and physicians' industries have indeed improved the quality of life for all Americans. However, by allowing huge pharmaceutical and insurance corporations with big lobbyists to have free rein to do as they wish to achieve greater profits at the expense of the people has brought the American health care system to its knees. Why not regulate these health care middlemen, who are jacking up the costs of health care to astronomical levels? Better yet, why not eliminate the insurance middlemen and save hundreds of billions of dollars with a national health care program that covers everyone equally? Is that such a socialist or revolutionary idea?

## WOULD A SINGLE-PAYER SYSTEM BE SO BAD?

Why can't we develop a single-payer plan for universal medical coverage, using the basic Medicare model? Imagine how much simpler life would be if we didn't have a hundred different insurance companies to be providers for, twenty different forms to submit our bills to, and twenty different prescription drug formularies to comply with when treating patients. Having lots of choices of health plans may seem like a good idea for employers or individual customers, but it is an absolute nightmare for physicians to be forced to adjust their treatments according to each of their individual patient's plans.

How would it be if the insurance companies could no longer control the cost and delivery of health care, and physicians were paid the same amount for all patients equally? How would it be for businesses not to have the sole burden of providing health care insurance to their employees at exorbitant rates? We could get all Americans covered, perhaps with a sliding-scale insurance premium based on income and some employer contributions. Everyone would and should be required to pay something for their health care, which would help to keep the value of their health in mind.

In a survey of 2193 physicians, 59% supported a single payer, national health insurance plan (Carroll, Aaron) Multiple public surveys, including a 2007 survey of 1821 adults have shown that approximately 65% felt that the United States should adopt a universal health insurance program in which everyone is covered under a program like Medicare that is run by the government and financed by taxpayers. (public ap/yahoo)

The fact is, we are paying more for our health care as a nation, by far, and getting much less. We are leaving over 50 million without insurance and many more with inadequate coverage. It is estimated that we could save approximately $400 billion and cover everyone by switching to a national health care plan. (Woolhandler, Steffie, 2002)

The amount of paperwork involved in caring for patients would be dramatically reduced. The headaches of trying to get authorization from various insurance companies for radiology or other testing, surgery, medications, or treatments could be streamlined such that a physician's order can be accompanied by the medical record and outliers can be peer-reviewed by a panel of physicians and subject to one standard of medical care, not hundreds of different standards or policy rules. This would free up time for physicians and their office staff to do what they were trained to do, to see more patients and provide them the best care they can. The insurance middlemen who are driving up the costs of health care so dramatically would be eliminated and some of those health care dollars freed up to reimburse physicians for being the foundation and driving force of health care, as they should be.

# A NATIONAL MALPRACTICE/ COMPLICATIONS FUND

One of the major areas that is draining the economy and the ability of physicians to practice medicine as they were trained is fear of liability and the practice of defensive medicine. In order for any other measures to take effect in controlling health care costs, we must change the system whereby physicians are sued for mistakes or errors that lead to complications in our patients.

Oversight of medical care and quality control could be handled by a physician's panel of peer reviewers with an outcomes, evidence-based set of guidelines that would bring some standardization to the practice of medicine without exerting too much control over the individual physician or stifling the creativity that comes from thinking outside the box or tailoring a treatment to fit the complex set of conditions in an individual patient. This could be a world where the threat of malpractice litigation does not loom over each physician's head, while at the same time there is some compensation for those who have an unexpected poor outcome due to a physician's mistake or negligence. It must be recognized that the vast majority of bad outcomes are related to years of abuse and neglect on the part of the patient, not the physician's efforts to reverse the ravages of time or to intervene in the natural course of events. Caps on awards and fines for frivolous lawsuits would help limit many lawsuits that are putting good physicians out of business today and discouraging others from entering the practice of medicine. By eliminating some of the bureaucracy and the obstacles, we would allow physicians time to do what they do best, practice their healing skills as they were trained to do.

Changes in health care must be both on a national level and on an individual level. The overall medical climate in which physicians practice, as well as individual relationships, must be addressed. The emotional bond between doctor and patient has been so heavily eroded in the current system of medicine that trust and communication are becoming a thing of the past. When physicians see each patient with a potential malpractice lawsuit in mind, we see ourselves as defendants rather than as allies in the battle against death and disease. We stop using our medical judgment based on history, examination, and differential diagnosis and start worrying about the outliers and rare diagnosis we could be missing, when ordering tests or treatments. In order to supplement their income, physicians may have ownership status in the radiology testing facility that they send their patients to, which gives them a financial incentive to order more unnecessary tests. The open, trusting relationship that was a foundation of the doctor-patient relationship allowed a physician to say, "This is probably nothing serious, let's try some medicine before we order a CT scan or MRI. If you are no better in a couple of weeks, we will reevaluate you. Call me if anything worsens." Now this is too risky, and in the five minutes you have to evaluate a patient, it is easier to order the extra tests on the initial evaluation and not take a chance. The patient may go home and suffer a complication, not come back or go to another doctor who makes a different diagnosis by ordering that expensive test first. Patients can and do sue physicians for less than that. Physicians know that just one lawsuit could destroy them. The standards of care are written for the majority of people with a given symptom or diagnosis and do not take into account the rare and atypical cases we as physicians frequently see. The standards are written by our specialty societies, shaped by research on the specified condition, and taught in our medical schools, yet occasionally we need to have the leeway to step outside the boundaries in order to make a brilliant diagnosis in the rare case. In addition, not all conditions are that well studied, and there are many gaps in these standards of care. There is a lack of interest and a lack of funding on the part of university research programs to evaluate treatments that do not have a payoff for some pharmaceutical company or equipment manufacturer. As government-funded research grants dry up, the only dollars out there are offered by the pharmaceutical companies, but not for pure, altruistic reasons. They want the outcome to involve a new medicine for which they can charge big money. It took the VA hospitals to perform large randomized trials to determine that aspirin was beneficial in prevention of stroke and heart disease, and many alternative, natural remedies will never be studied thoroughly because no one can make much of a profit on an herb that can be purchased or grown without a prescription. The risk for physicians who incorporate alternative treatments into their practices is great, and the benefits small. Yet a few physicians are doing it because we have seen empirically that they work. A new era of health care must incorporate preventative and alternative medicine and support for research that is not influenced by the big pharmaceutical drug companies.

Remember that physicians are human beings, and we do make mistakes in treating patients, some of which cause irreparable harm to our patients. However, frivolous law suits against doctors must come to an end. Despite a physician's best efforts, poor outcomes inevitably do happen, and a lawsuit isn't going to change anything except to line the pockets of one individual and his or her lawyer, while raising the cost of health care for all. Not all malpractice lawsuits are inappropriate, but unless there is a pattern of willful negligence, lawsuits are simply ineffective at improving a physician's doctoring skills or knowledge. Physicians are not and never will be perfect, especially with the added pressure to see more and more patients in less time. It is impossible to keep up entirely with the rapidly expanding base of knowledge in every field of medicine. Unrealistic demands and expectations are overwhelming physicians and causing them to get out of the practice of medicine.

What can we do to help out those patients who suffer severe complications of treatment or those who are truly victims of malpractice? What if we were to set up a trust fund to make reparations to those patients who suffer complications of treatments by physicians who have made a mistake or even committed malpractice? This could be achieved without requiring that a lawsuit be filed, would have caps on how much money one could receive for one's injuries, provide for future medical care, and would have physician oversight and a review board that could actually get to the root of the problem with physicians who have a track record of frequent complications or negligence. It could be similar to workers' compensation, where instead of paying exorbitant malpractice insurance premiums each year, physicians would contribute to this trust fund, which would be invested until it is needed. This would also allow for greater self-policing of physicians by physicians, and provide a mechanism for specific additional training for physicians when a pattern of complications is identified. It would eliminate the risk of that physician losing everything, including their careers, because of a single lawsuit. Medical review boards are not a new concept and are already in place in hospitals and on panels of various insurance companies and medical management companies. They are already a part of state licensing boards. If these groups were working together to form a coalition with a single set of standards or guidelines, it would allow physicians to police themselves more effectively. Without the risk of malpractice lawyers having access to physicians' records and using them against an individual physician in court, it would improve the quality of health care in this country for all.

Most hospital review boards are essentially impotent when it comes to dealing effectively with a negligent physician because of the medico-legal risks involved and the fear that some lawyer will get hold of the documents associated with these review boards. We need to empower those review boards already in place and set up guidelines such that every physician has a clear understanding of the guidelines by which they are judged. Responsibility on a personal and professional level must be the main priority, including the conservation of health care resources, regardless of who is footing the bill—insurance companies, individuals, or the government. Fiscal responsibility is something that is often at odds with the current health care system, where everyone is trying to carve out a portion of the health care dollars being spent. If you were in charge of an island of people with very limited resources and had no choice but to prioritize the delivery of that care, you would find ways to cut back on unnecessary tests and treatments that were not shown to be effective or to improve the quality of life. We have to start thinking that way, and in the long run this is will lead to the best quality of health care at lower cost for our patients as well.

*Diana Reed, M.D.*

# PHYSICIANS AND PATIENTS:
# HEAL YOUR HEALTH CARE SYSTEM

I believe that physicians need to have the authority returned to them to practice medicine as they were trained. They need to be allowed to prescribe tests and treatments as they see fit for each individual patient. Physicians need to have their hands cut loose from the restraints imposed by insurance companies and government regulators in their day-to-day activities. We need to be allowed to practice medicine equally for all patients, without first having to consider what insurance plan they are covered by. This would eliminate the caste system we currently have, which is based on the insurance plans that individual patients have or whether they even have health insurance. Insurance plans need to have one list of benefits that determines whether diagnostic tests, surgery, and other treatments or medications will be covered. Simplification is the key to survival for physicians and to saving health care dollars and lives in the long run.

Everyone wants people to be able to choose his or her own doctors, whether they are primary care or specialty physicians. If all practicing physicians were covered as providers under a nationwide plan, patients could choose their physicians without financial penalties. We want our patients to come to us because they want us to treat them, not because some insurance company says they must. Sometimes our patients' personality differences attract them to one or another physician. Patients also have different expectations of how a physician should be. It may have little to do with the skill or knowledge a physician possesses; each physician has a unique personality and practice style. If patients are not forced to switch from one physician to another as their insurance coverage changes, they have a chance to bond with their doctor and get to know them. They become more comfortable discussing their health and the most personal issues they face. Their doctors, over time, get to know their patients better. They take into account the nuances of their medical condition and their individual personalities, as they choose a treatment plan tailored to their patients. They become more than doctor and patient, they become friends and allies in the most significant struggle people face during their lives, the battle against their own mortality.

If there is mutual trust and compassion between doctor and patient, the rates of success in overcoming illness rise dramatically. In all medical

162

research studies, patients given a placebo by a caring, compassionate physician can get well from even the most serious illness, if they believe in their treatment and have faith in their doctor to help them get well. Up to thirty percent of patients in a research study will benefit from a placebo, even though there is no active medication in it. This is why double-blind studies are considered the best standard to determine whether a medication is really effective. It must be more effective than the placebo effect of faith and trust. There is tremendous power in the mind and its ability to cure the body it inhabits. When there is a sense of hope and a strong belief in the physician and the treatment, amazing things can happen, which are well beyond the boundaries of known science. Good physicians know this, and make use of the intangible healing abilities of faith every day, as do many other healers in alternative medicine and religious fields. The combination of good science and faith are even more powerful than either one alone, and this has been proven in scientific studies. To achieve the best in health care, there must be a relationship between doctor and patient that fosters faith and the belief that healing will take place. Doctors really don't want to play God, but it doesn't hurt to bring Him into the healing process.

All physicians want to remove the financial obstacles to delivering the best-quality health care in all our communities. We are tired and frustrated at having to stratify the health care according to our patients' insurance coverage or lack thereof. Some form of national health care with a single-payer system would allow physicians to provide care for their patients equally, as we were trained to do, without having to turn some away because of their inability to pay. We would no longer have to make choices about who gets which medication, test, or treatment based on their insurance coverage. Patients and physicians could only benefit from these changes. We need to enact some real reform in the system that places the emphasis where it belongs—on doctors and their patients, and on the health and well-being of the entire American population. There has been a bill, HR676, introduced by Representative John Conyers which would provide health care as expanded Medicare benefits with a single payer that has been languishing in Congress, and getting killed in committee that could save $400 billion while providing health care to all. If our lawmakers would listen to the people that elected them instead of the big corporate powers, they would know that the majority of Americans in multiple surveys want national health care. There are ways in which we as Americans can change the downward spiral of our health care system, and there is always hope for the future. Physicians need to take the responsibility to be leaders in navigating those changes; the government and the people need to help us bring those changes about.

As an American, I believe in capitalism and the right to make a profit from one's career. Physicians, however are held to different standards than other businesses and are restricted on both the income and expense sides of the economic equation. As the costs of health care have risen steadily, physicians have seen significant reductions in their income in the past several years. However, other organizations involved in providing health care to our citizens are reaping huge profits at the expense of the people, and the legal profession is driving the costs of health care to astronomical proportions. The medical field is unlike any other business, and human values need to come before profits. The current system is not living up to that standard, while physicians and patients suffer. It is difficult to understand how health insurance executives should make fifteen million dollar annual salaries and bonuses, while physicians on the front lines do the work of providing medical care to the population.

Physicians may not be the best businessmen; we want to put our patients' health first, regardless of cost considerations. It is a sad fact that physicians have given up control of our field to the powerful insurance companies, pharmaceuticals, and the government. We have become pawns in the field of medicine to be controlled and pushed in directions that don't make U.S. health care the best—only the most expensive and administratively complicated. Small groups of people, CEOs, insurance executives, and administrative middlemen are walking away with millions or even billions of dollars that are desperately needed to keep our whole population healthy. If we could get rid of the middlemen, there would be doctors and patients, lower hospital and medication costs and better-quality health care. To achieve such a goal, patients and doctors need to come together. We need to pressure our congressmen to stop listening to the powerful lobbyists of the insurance companies, managed care companies, the pharmaceutical companies, and the trial lawyers. We need to enact some real reform in the system that places the emphasis where it belongs, on the doctor and their patients, and the health and well-being of the entire American population.

I feel that we must hold these medical middlemen accountable. Insurance companies, pharmaceuticals, and managed care organizations must accept their portion of the burden for health care, which is now squarely on the backs of doctors and their patients. They are profit-driven companies, and the provision of health care should not be based on one's ability to pay or being disease free. Unregulated, these companies will continue to raise prices, provide less, and leave more and more Americans in the cold.

Physicians spend half of their lives training for their careers and go deeply into debt to pay for that training. They sacrifice any chance at a normal life without beepers, long hours, and ongoing responsibility for thousands of their patients. They devote themselves to improving this world, one patient at a time. However, there has been a deep dissatisfaction brewing among physicians, which is causing many physicians to quit the practice of medicine. If we don't encourage the physicians we have to stay with it, and encourage potential physicians to take on the required years of training, we will all suffer when the predicted shortages of physicians becomes a reality.

Why would anyone want to be a physician? Every day we deal with serious illnesses, most of which are still incurable, despite many advances in the field of medicine. As we hold the hands of people with diseases like cancer, stroke, heart disease, diabetes, and degenerative illnesses, we face the reality of our own imperfection. Often, we are up to our eyeballs in urine, feces, vomit and blood, as we risk our own health in the service of others. While we are unable to relieve our patients completely from their medical problems, we do help our patients manage their conditions and provide support as they struggle to conquer their pain and suffering. As we try to keep our patients' health and wellness in mind, we must also maintain our awareness that every patient we see is a potential lawsuit, regardless of our actions or the quality of our medical care. At the same time that we empathize and care for our patients individually, we must keep an eye on the clock ticking and the next patient in the waiting room. Instead of sitting for a while to listen to an old man tell stories of his past, we are now pressured to move on to the next patient. If we don't squeeze enough patients into each day, we will find ourselves going out of business.

In times of sickness and in worldwide disasters, who do we turn to when we face our own mortality? We assume that doctors will always be there for their patients. Will patients always be there for their doctors? Will America come to the aid of their physicians, in their time of need?

Patients, talk to your doctors, ask them how they are doing with their health care business, and how the new legislation will affect their practices.

Open the lines of communication, and you might be surprised at the responses you get. Show some compassion and understanding for the stress that physicians are under during these difficult times.

As we face the current crisis in health care, will patients rally to support legislation that will limit the power of the managed care middlemen who are restricting the ability of physicians to treat their patients as they see fit? Will they help enact legislation that will limit the awards given in malpractice suits, punish lawyers who file multiple frivolous lawsuits, and thereby help to reduce insurance premiums? Will they help put pressure on pharmaceutical companies to make drugs affordable for everyone, whether they have prescription coverage or not? Will they stop the extortion of Americans to pay for the huge profits enjoyed by pharmaceutical corporations, and limit price-fixing and loopholes preventing cheaper generic drugs from becoming available, before they bankrupt the nation?

If we are to turn the health care crisis around, we must make several major policy changes at once. I believe that, in order to be effective, there should be a tripod of basic health insurance for all with a single national rate plan, malpractice litigation reform with a national compensation fund for patients with poor outcomes related to medical errors, headed up by a board of physician specialists, and finally, the freedom for physicians to practice medicine as they were trained, with patients who choose them of their own free will. Physicians would be given the choice of a salaried position or fee for service reimbursement. Blue collar workers, physicians, lawyers, corporate CEO's, the handicapped and the mentally ill, government workers would finally achieve the civilized status of equality at the most basic, life and death level. When you need to go to a doctor, you go. No co-pays, coinsurance, deductibles or denials to worry about when making a decision about your health or that of your family. The Medicare tax we already pay would need to be revised and everyone able to work would pay a percentage of their income. There would be no profit motive so administrative costs could be kept to a minimum, as the Medicare and VA systems already have shown.

These changes would help simplify the paperwork mountains that physicians are buried in, ease their fears of malpractice litigation, and restore dignity and control of medical decision making back to where it belongs—in the sacred relationship between the doctor and his or her patient. Patients and physicians, heal thyselves and thy health care system!

# AFTERWORD

Since completion of this book, I joined a group called Physicians for a National Healthcare Program, or PNHP. I attended their annual meeting in Washington DC, and was amazed at the dedication and credentials of the leaders in this movement. Their activism for equality in health care is truly inspiring.

In the fall of 2011, a new movement had sprung up called Occupy. It started with Occupy Wall Street, with a group of people that camped out in front of the New York Stock Exchange to protest corporate greed, corporate personhood, and the influence of the 1% over our governments elected officials and legislation. From the physicians' standpoint, corporate greed is killing our patients and our profession, and is a perfect example of how badly broken the current system is. What we have is wealth care, not health care in this country.

PNHP decided to officially support the Occupy Wall Street Movement, and did so by getting directly involved, providing a first aid/medical presence in the encampments, as well as carrying signs and even getting arrested along with others for their non-violent protests. Dr Margaret Flowers has led the charge in Occupy Washington DC, and encouraged all of us physicians to get involved.

I came home from this meeting full of excitement and hope about the future of medicine. It was a feeling I had not had for a long time. I got involved in my local chapter, Occupy Nashville, and have helped to get some first aid supplies, vitamins and food. Together with donations and help from others, we were able to get a medical tent set up, flu shots for the people camping out on Legislative Plaza, and patch up the occasional cuts, bruises or colds people developed out in the elements. I helped to obtain flu shots, tetanus vaccines and tuberculosis screening for the people in our encampment. I also found myself adopting this group as my small flock of patients, volunteering my time to promote a national health care plan that would cover everyone, regardless of their station in life. I saw firsthand the desperate need for mental health care and substance abuse treatment in our forgotten homeless population that struggle each day to survive on the streets. Although I am physically unable to camp out with these dedicated young people, I consider myself a part time Occupier, and definitely in the 99%.

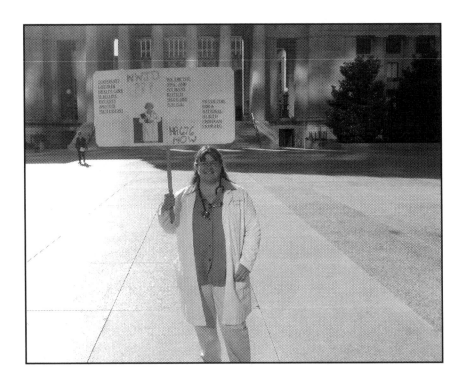

# BIBLIOGRAPHY

Smith, Mark, Mosley, Kurt, Schaumburg, Steve, Godwin, Stephanie, Autry, Chad. The Physicians' Foundation. "The Physicians Perspective Medical Practice in 2008(survey summary and analysis)," Merritt Hawkins & Associates August 25, 2008.

Croasdale, Myrle. "Federal Advisory Group Predicts Physician Shortage Looming." *American Medical Association News,* November 3, 2003.

Association of American Medical Colleges US Medical School Applicants and Students 1982–83 to 2010–11 http://www.aamc.org/facts October 2010 accessed September 13, 2011

Dyrbye, Liselotte N., Thomas, Matthew R., Massie, F. Stanford, Power, David V., Eaker, Annie, Harper, William, Durning, Steven, Moutier, Christine M., Szydio, Daniel W., Novotny, Paul J., Sloan, Jeff A., Shanafelt, Tait D. "Burnout and Suicidal Ideation among U.S. Medical Students." *Annals of Internal Medicine* 149, no. 5 (September 2, 2008):334–341.

American College of Physicians. "Residency Match Results Not Encouraging for Adults Needing Primary Care." News Release, March 18, 2010. http://www.acponline.org/pressroom/residency_match.htm Accessed October 12, 2011

Merritt, Hawkins and Associates. "Survey Report 2003 Survey of Final-Year Medical Residents." Irving, Tx.: Merritt, Hawkins & Associates 2003. www.merritthawkins.com Accessed February 3, 2005

Kaiser Family Foundation. "National Survey of Physicians, Part III: Doctors' Opinions about Their Profession, 2002." Menlo Park, Ca: The Henry J. Kaiser Family Foundation. March 2002 www.kff.org Accessed October 2, 2005

Adams, Damon. "Physicians Are Working More, Enjoying It Less." *American Medical Association News,* June 3, 2002.

Kilani, R. K., Paxton, B. E., Stinnett, S. S., Barnhart, H. X., Bindal, V., & Lungren, M. P. "Self-Referral in Medical Imaging: A Meta-Analysis of the Literature." Journal of the American College of Radiology. 8, no. 7 (2011):469–76.

Merritt, Hawkins and Associates. Year 2000 Survey of Physicians 50 Years Old and Older. Irving, Tx. Merritt Hawkins & Associates April 2000 www.merritthawkins.com Accessed September 24, 2005

Merritt, Hawkins and Associates. Year 2004 Survey of Physicians 50 to 65 Years Old. Irving, Tx. Merritt, Hawkins & Associates Irving, Tx. 2004 www.merritthawkins.com Accessed Sept 24, 2005

Wikipedia.org. "Gabapentin." Accessed Sept. 14, 2011.

Beasley, Deena, & Hirschler, Ben. "Ending Drug Companies'Addiction to Price Rises." Medscape.com/viewarticle/742661. Accessed May 12, 2011.

Nelson, Roxanne. "Drug Shortages Predicted to Reach Record Levels." Medscape.com/viewarticle/749401. Accessed September 9, 2011.

Salahi, Lara. "Obama Issues Executive Order to Ease Drug Shortages." ABC News October 31, 2011. http://abcnews.go.com/Health/Wellness/presidents-executive-order-drug-shortage-draws-mixed-reactions/story?id=14852829 Accessed Nov. 18, 2011

Hoffman, James M., Shah, Nilay D., Vermeulen, Lee C., Doloresco, Fred. Martin, Patrick K., Blake, Sharon, Matusiak, Linda, Hunkler, Robert J., & Schumock, Glen T. "Projecting Future Drug Expenditures—2009." *American Journal of Health-System Pharmacy* 66 (February 1, 2009):237–257.

Ismail, M. Asif. "Drug Lobby Second to None—How the Pharmaceutical

Industry Gets Its Way in Washington." (Special Report). The Center for Public Integrity, 2005.

Dilanian, Ken. "Senators Who Weakened Drug Bill Got Millions From Industry." *USA Today*, May 11, 2007.

Mercer, Lisa Marie. "List of Companies Outsourcing Pharmacy Work to India." www.livestrong.com/article/26195. Accessed October 15, 2009.

Crane, Mark. "20% Error Rate in Processing Claims, AMA Study Finds." Medscape Medical News. www.medscape.com/viewarticle745041. Accessed June 21, 2011.

Hellinger, Fred J., & Encinosa, William E. "Impact of State Laws Limiting Malpractice Awards on Geographic Distribution of Physicians." U.S. Dept. of Health and Human Services Agency for Healthcare Research and Quality, 2002.

*CNN Money*. "Fortune 500 Top Industries: Most Profitable," May 5, 2008. http://www.money.cnn.com/magazines/fortune/fortune500/2008/performers/industries Accessed September 19, 2011

U.S. Census Bureau. "Income, Poverty and Health Insurance Coverage in the United States," 2010.

Mayne, Lorraine, Girod, Chris, & Weltz, Scott. "Healthcare Costs for American Families Double in Less Than Nine Years." Milliman Medical Index. 2011. http://insight.milliman.com. Accessed May 11, 2011.

Wilper, Andrew, Woolhandler, Steffie, Lasser, Karen, McCormick, Danny, Bor, David, Himmelstein, David "Health Insurance and Mortality in US Adults." *American Journal of Public Health* 99:12 December 2009

Wilper, Andrew, Woolhandler, Steffie, Lasser Karen, McCormick, Danny, Bor, David, Himmelstein, David. "A National Study of Chronic Disease Prevalence and Access to Care in Uninsured U.S. Adults." *Annals of Internal Medicine* 149:3 August 5, 2008 170-176

Tamkins, Theresa. "Medical Bills Prompt More Than 60 Percent of U.S. Bankruptcies."

*CNN Health*, June 5, 2009.

Greene, Jay. "Physicians Enticed into Early Retirement." *American Medical Association News*, July 24, 2000.

Iglehart, John. "Health Reform, Primary Care and Graduate Medical Education."

*New England Journal of Medicine* 363 (August 5, 2010):584–590.

Agency for HealthCare Research and Quality Patient Safety and Quality. "Doctors are Willing to Report and Learn From Medical Mistakes, but Find Error-Reporting Systems Inadequate." July, 2008.

Patient Protection and Affordable Care Act HR03590, March 23, 2010.

Health Reform and the Decline of Physician Private Practice: A White Paper

The Physicians Foundation. "Examining the Effects of the Patient Protection and Affordable Care Act on Physician Practices in the United States," October, 2008.

Jacob, Julie A. "Losing Proposition: When Doctors Take in Less Than What Goes Out." *American Medical Association News*, January 7, 2002.

Steiger, Bill. "Discouraged Doctors Survey Results: Doctors Say Morale Is Hurting." (Special Report). ACPE Tool Kit on Physician Morale, January 10, 2007.

Cohen, Duffie. Survey of Young Physicians on Establishing their Careers and Providing Care in the Changing Medical Marketplace (1987–1997), Robert Wood Johnson Foundation Princeton, N.J. updated June 2000. http://www.rwjf.org/reports/grr/028326s.htm Accessed November 3, 2003

National Practitioner Data Bank Annual Reports, 2000 and 2006. Dept. of Health and Human Services Health Resources and Services Administration Bureau of Health Professions Division of Practitioner Data Banks http://www.npdb-hipdb.hrsa.gov/annualrpt.html Accessed Sept. 24 2007

Towers Watson Report. "2010 Update on U.S. Tort Costs Trends," Appendix 5, "Medical Malpractice Tort Cost Trends." http://www. towerswatson.com. Accessed Sept. 24, 2011

"Defensive Medicine among High-Risk Specialist Physicians in a Volatile

Malpractice Environment" (abstract), *Journal of the American Medical Association*,

293 (2005):2609–2617.

Jena, Anupam, Seabury, Seth, Lakdawalla, Darius, & Chandra, Amitabh. "Malpractice Risk According to Physician Specialty." *New England Journal of Medicine*, 365 (August 18, 2011):629–636.

Stuudert, David M., Mello, Michelle, Gawande, Atul, Gandhi, Tejal, Kachalia, Allen

Yoon, Catherine, Puopolo, Ann, & Brennan, Troyen. Claims, Errors, and Compensation Payments in Medical Malpractice Litigation. *New England Journal of Medicine*, 354 (May 11, 2006), no. 19:2024–2033.

Todd, Heather Lasher. "New AMA Report Finds 95 Medical Liability Claims Filed For Every 100 Physicians." *American Medical Association News*, August 3, 2010.

Florida Medical Malpractice Insurance History 2000–2010.

http://www.mymedicalmalpracticeinsurance.com Accessed August 29, 2011

Merritt Hawkins and Associates Summary Report 2003: Obstetrics/ Gynecology Malpractice Survey. Irving, Tx. Merritt, Hawkins & Associates 2003 www.merritthawkins.com Accessed Sept 24, 2005

Mello, Michelle M., Studdert, David M., Des Roches, Catherine M., Peugh, Jordan, Zapert, Kinga, Brennan, Troyen A., & Sage, William M. "Caring for Patients in a Malpractice Crisis: Physician Satisfaction and Quality of Care." *Health Affairs* 23(2004), no. 4: 42–53.

Institute of Medicine Committee on Quality of Health Care in America.

"To Err is Human: Building a Safer Health System." Washington, D.C.: National Academy Press, 2000.

Copland, James R. "A Report on the Lawsuit Industry in America, 2003A Message from the Director." Trial Lawyers, Inc. Center for Legal Policy, Manhattan Institute for Policy Research, 2003. http://triallawyersinc. com/html/print01.html Accessed Nov 17,2011

Tanner, Michael D. "The Grass is Not Always Greener: A Look at National Health Care Systems Around the World." Medscape Connect, http:// boards.medscape.com/forums?14@@.29ebf99d.29ebf99c Accessed November 15, 2008.

White, Andrew, Gallagher, Thomas, Krauss, Melissa, Garbutt, Jane, Waterman, Amy, Dunagan, Claiborne, Fraser, Victoria, Levinson, Wendy, & Larson, Eric. "The Attitudes and Experiences of Trainees Regarding Disclosing Medical Errors to

Patients." *Academic Medicine*, 83(2008), no. 3:250–256.

Albert, Tanya. Physicians Feel Double Digit Pain as Liability Rates Continue to Rise. *American Medical Association News,* November 10, 2003.

Slepian, Lauren. "Americans Believe Access to Health Care Threatened by Medical Liability Crisis." Wirthlin Worldwide, 2003 Health Coalition on Liability and Access. http://www.hcla.org Accessed Sept. 24, 2005

Hellinger, Fred E., & Encinosa, William E. "Review of Reforms to our Medical Liability System." U.S. Dept. of Health and Human Services Agency for Healthcare Research and Quality, December 31, 2009.

Lowes, Robert. "Regional Variation in Malpractice Premiums Defies Tort Reform."

www.medscape.com/viewarticle/731833. Accessed November 2, 2010.

Americans for Insurance Reform. "Medical Malpractice Insurance: Stable Losses/Unstable Rates." New York, NY. March 28, 2007.

Ubel, Peter, Angott, Andrea, Zikmund-Fisher, Brian. "Physicians Recommend Different Treatments for Patients Than They Would

Choose for Themselves." *Arch Intern Med.* 171(7):630-634 April 11, 2011

Durand, Bryan. "Nation's Frontline Physicians Unhappy with Healthcare Reform Measures." The Physicians Foundation November 18, 2010

Carroll, Aaron. "Support for National Health Insurance among U.S. Physicians: 5 Years Later." *Annals of Internal Medicine* 148:7;566 April 2008

"In December 2007, 65 percent of Americans supported a "universal health insurance program in which everyone is covered under a program like Medicare that is run by the government and financed by taxpayers." Associated Press–Yahoo Poll, 14–20 December 2007, http://news.yahoo.com/page/election-2008-political-pulse-voter-worries Accessed 30 January 2008

Woolhandler, Steffie, Himmelstein, David. "Paying for National Health Insurance—and Not Getting It," *Health Affairs* 21, no. 4 (2002): 88–98.

# INDEX

## A

Accountable Care Organization 149
AIDS 51, 152
Allopathic medicine 68
Alternative medicine 40, 68, 69, 160, 163
American Medical Association 74, 106, 114, 169, 170, 172–174
Americans for Insurance Reform 124, 174
anxiety 31, 34, 35, 38, 43, 85, 86, 125, 136, 137
Arbitration 82
art of medicine 13, 46, 98
attending physician 14, 15, 17, 24, 66, 127, 128, 137
Attorneys 103, 107, 114

## B

B12 deficiency 112
back pain 35, 37, 54, 139, 141
Bad patients 48, 49
Blue Cross 81, 82
Board certification 22
brain tumor 35, 36, 79, 125
Business of medicine ix, 4, 22, 29, 41, 57, 90

## C

Capitated managed care 59
Center for Medicare and Medicaid Services 94
CEOs 64, 71, 102, 148, 164
Cerebral palsy 109
Cesarean section 121
chronic back pain 35
Clinical trials 40, 62, 69
Cobra 78, 79
Collateral source rule 122
Collective bargaining 5, 73, 96, 97
Compliance 49, 53, 92, 113, 135, 149
Complications 39, 69, 105, 108, 113, 117, 118, 121, 122, 127, 128, 133, 135–138, 154, 158, 160, 161
concierge practices 103
Corporate greed 148, 167
Council on Graduate Medical Education 86

# M

malpractice  ix, 4, 5, 7, 23, 31, 50, 56, 61, 73, 75, 76, 86, 87, 89–91, 99,
  104–108, 110, 111, 114–124, 130, 131, 133, 134, 155, 158–161, 166,
  171, 173, 174
malpractice claims  4, 89, 105, 106, 115, 118
malpractice crisis  173
malpractice insurance  61, 75, 76, 91, 107, 114–116, 118–120, 121–124, 130,
  161, 173, 174
malpractice lawsuits  7, 31, 76, 90, 91, 106, 108, 110, 114, 120, 160
malpractice liability  75, 76, 89, 115, 118
malpractice litigation  114, 158, 166, 173
managed care  ix, 23, 35, 41, 46, 48, 54, 56, 58–60, 62, 77, 78, 80, 81, 83, 85,
  86, 89, 96, 102, 124, 148, 153, 154, 164, 166
Mandatory reporting laws  33
Marketing  63, 64, 66, 70
MCAT  10, 11
Medicaid  60, 61, 73, 81, 84, 94, 96, 97, 100, 103, 110, 148, 149
MediCal  ix, x, 3, 4, 5, 7, 9, 11–27, 29, 31, 34, 38–43, 46–49, 51–53, 56, 57,
  59–62, 66, 68–71, 73, 74, 76, 78, 80–84, 85–92, 96, 98–101, 103–108,
  110, 111, 113–115, 118–120, 122, 123, 125, 128, 131–133, 135, 136,
  140, 143, 146–148, 150–162, 164–167, 169–174
medical bills  7, 84, 103, 171
medical equipment  91
Medical errors  118, 119, 131, 150, 154, 166, 174
Medical mistakes  118, 150, 172
Medical school  ix, 4, 9, 11–14, 16, 18–20, 21, 24–26, 38, 39, 60, 68, 69, 80,
  82, 108, 135, 143, 151, 159, 169
Medical school applicants  169
Medical societies  83
Medical specialties  17, 18
Medical student  12, 17–21, 25, 26, 100, 136, 169
Medical supplies  103
Medicare  33, 37, 47, 55, 61, 64, 71–73, 83, 84, 91, 93–95, 96, 97, 100, 102,
  103, 110, 148, 149, 157, 163, 166, 175
Medicare audits  95
Medicare Fee Schedule  95
Medicare Part D  64, 71
Medicare Volume Performance Standards (MVPS)  95
Medico-legal system  113
Mental illness  39, 42, 52
Merritt, Hawkins and Associates  19, 22, 56, 86, 169, 170
Micromanagement  78, 83, 149, 153
Middlemen  62, 102, 156–158, 164, 166
Migraine  18, 34, 36, 66, 67, 125

Milliman Medical Index  84, 171
MRI scan  33, 37, 47, 85, 109, 125
multiple sclerosis  20, 72
Multispecialty groups  ix, 58, 75
Myasthenia gravis  82
Myelogram  109

## N

National Practitioner Data Bank  106, 172
Neurology  ix, 17, 20, 23, 31, 32, 37, 40, 51, 57, 60, 66, 69, 72, 94, 96, 97,
    109, 112, 131–133, 137, 145
Neurontin  63
Neuroradiologist  126–128, 132
Neurosurgery  20, 36, 74, 75, 91, 113, 115, 123, 133
New England Journal of Medicine  106, 172, 173
Nursing home regulations  108

## O

oath for doctors of medicine  21, 27
Obama health care plan  148
Obstetrics and gynecology  16
Occupy Nashville  167
Occupy Wall Street  167
Occupy Washington DC  167
Omnibus Budget Reconciliation Act of 1989  95
Ophthalmologist  59, 60

## P

Pain clinics  50
Paperwork  4, 7, 30, 35, 41, 43, 46, 58, 77, 79, 80, 83, 102, 103, 108, 137,
    148, 149, 152, 158, 166
Patent laws  63
Patents  64, 129
Patient Protection and Affordable Care Act  x, 101, 148, 172
Pfizer  63
Pharmaceutical advertising  70
Pharmaceutical companies  6, 62–69, 70–72, 83, 102, 120, 155, 160, 164, 166
Pharmaceutical industry  54, 64, 67, 170
physician extenders  98, 104
physician morale  172
Pimping  17
Placebo  66–69, 151, 163
Plasmapheresis  82
PPO  81, 100

practice of medicine  12, 29, 41, 75, 88, 100, 146, 155, 158–160, 165

Practice of medicine  12, 29, 41, 75, 88, 100, 146, 155, 158–160, 165

Pregnancy  108, 121, 136

Prescriptions  40, 41, 44, 47, 50, 79, 103, 149, 150, 154

primary care physician  79, 111, 112

Private practice  ix, 3, 4, 19, 23, 29, 44, 57, 60, 61, 75, 80, 92, 93, 98, 100, 141, 149, 172

Profit margins  83, 156

Provider  5, 58, 59, 73–76, 78, 79, 81, 83–85, 87, 93, 96, 97, 116, 123, 157, 162

Pseudomeningocele  142

pseudoseizure  38

Psychiatry  16, 18, 20, 39, 52, 94, 96, 98

Psychological  13, 31, 34, 38, 39, 52–54

Punitive damages  115, 155

## Q

Quality health care  81, 88, 89, 102, 106, 156, 163, 164

## R

radiology managed care  ix, 78, 148, 153

Radiology testing  54, 79, 87, 159

rebound headaches  35, 141

rehabilitation  32, 109, 120

Relative Value Units  94

Research  11, 18, 19, 24, 62, 69–71, 87, 100, 103, 151–153, 159, 160, 163, 171, 172, 174

Research grants  100, 160

residency  ix, 12, 16, 18–23, 29, 66, 69, 80, 144, 169

Rule of joint and severable liability  122

## S

Scut monkey  14

Seizures  34, 38, 110, 111

Shortages of physicians  104, 133, 147, 165

Standards of care  88, 155, 159, 160

Stethoscope  x, 4, 7, 22, 83, 145, 146

Stroke  18, 32, 33, 39, 40, 42, 112, 113, 120, 121, 126, 132, 160, 165

Student loan debt  19, 30

Student loans  19

surgeon  14, 40, 43, 50, 54, 58, 94, 129–131, 138–140, 142

surgery  x, 3, 6, 13, 16–19, 21, 25, 32, 35, 37, 43, 50, 54, 58, 59, 77, 79, 94, 97, 109–112, 115, 123, 125–127, 129, 130, 138, 139, 141–143, 154, 158, 162

# ABOUT THE AUTHOR

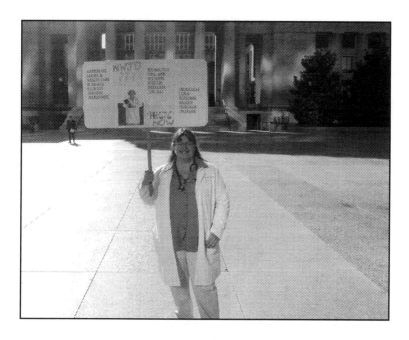

Dr. Diana Reed was born in New York, trained in California, attending UC–Irvine for medical school and UC–San Diego for her neurology residency. Dr. Reed had two children during medical school. She is a board-certified neurologist who has worked in five states, in solo private practice, small groups, and a large multispecialty group, as locum tenens, and as assistant professor at Vanderbilt University School of Medicine. She has been published in the *Journal of Surgical Pathology and Neurology* and has given numerous lectures. At the peak of her clinical career, she became disabled by complications of spine surgery but later recovered enough to work in radiology managed care. After five spine surgeries, she is now retired and lives near Nashville, Tennessee.

With a wide range of experience in medicine and personal health issues, she is able to reflect and report on the life of the physician and how the health care crisis is affecting physicians and patients. Her mission is to convey how important it is that all people pay attention to the medical profession and understand health care issues from the physician's perspective.